Overcoming Inflammatory Breast Cancer

Paul H. Levine, MD
Deborah D. Lange

Bethesda Communications Group

Published by the Bethesda Communications Group
4816 Montgomery Lane
Bethesda, MD 20814
www.bcgpub.com

ISBN-13: 978-1-7357729-0-5

Cover design, book design, and text editing by Deborah Lange

To the patients who have lived with inflammatory breast cancer, facing it with courage, determination, and creativity

Acknowledgments

Patti Bradfield inspired this book when she sent Deborah Lange six stories of women who had overcome inflammatory Breast Cancer (IBC) and had gone on to live healthy and productive lives. Patti envisioned an optimistic book about IBC in which doctors and patients alike recognize the symptoms of IBC, respond to it quickly with the latest treatments, and turn a once-deadly disease into a manageable chronic condition. This would be a sequel to her first book, *Nobody's Listening: Stories of inflammatory Breast Cancer*, which she wrote with Massimo Cristofanilli, MD, and which described IBC as a disease that often went unrecognized and misdiagnosed. Thank you Patti for being the catalyst to our endeavor.

As ideas began to percolate for our book, Paul H. Levine, MD, joined the effort and eventually took charge of the medical section, inviting other experts in the field to contribute also. Thank you Carmela Veneroso, MPH, Massimo Cristofanilli, MD, Ken Van Golen, PhD, Sangjucta Barkataki, PhD, Madhura Joglekar-Javadekar, PhD, Jennifer M. Rosenbluth, MD, PhD, Beth A. Overmoyer, MD, and Naoto T. Ueno, MD, PhD, for invaluable information about diagnostics, treatments, and research.

A heartfelt thank you to the patients who shared the stories of their journeys through this frightening disease: Nancy Key, Christine Paroz, Kathy Patton, Pat Shodean, Amy Pitman, Rosemary Heise, Jeannine Donahue, Vanetta Harrington, Anne K. Abate, Kim Alexander, Jenee Bobbora, and Amy Berman. You put a human face on an abstract medical diagnosis and show through your courage and creativity how to take command of difficult circumstances and not only make them work for you, but in many cases, give you strength and renewed purpose.

We are also grateful to Carmela Veneroso for reviewing the book and offering helpful comments.

And finally, thank you to The Inflammatory Breast Cancer Foundation (EraseIBC.org) for their generous support in helping us publish this book.

Paul H. Levine, MD, FACP, FACE
Deborah D. Lange

Contents

Foreword

This book is important to the IBC community and everyone who wants to learn about IBC. It contains medical facts about IBC and stories from patients. Because of the increased awareness of IBC, clinics dedicated to its treatment, and focused research programs in the US and abroad, we have witnessed an unprecedented improvement in survival rates for this disease that are of a larger magnitude than for other forms of breast cancer. While there are areas of epidemiology and early diagnosis that can further improve outcomes, for the first time our understanding of IBC is such that the future is brighter for IBC patients. We are grateful for the relentless work of dedicated researchers.

Cancer research in general has made tremendous strides in discovering major risk factors, both genetic and environmental. By describing the underlining molecular mechanisms, research has contributed to understanding drug resistance and has brought forth the development of novel, tailored prevention and treatment strategies, resulting in improved quality of life and improved outcomes.

Breast cancer is among the most predictable diseases in risk factors, patterns of local and distant spread, and recurrence and subtype-specific response to treatments. It is recognized that breast cancer is not a single entity but a combination of diseases defined by molecular signatures at the genomic level together with ethnic and endocrine-related factors playing a role in defining clinical behavior.

Inflammatory breast cancer (IBC) does not typically fit any of the criteria we recognize for malignancies and breast cancer. For reasons mainly still unknown, IBC spreads quickly to the breast lymphatics, and it affects young women that may not have any specific risk factors.

The Inflammatory Breast Cancer International Consortium (IBC-IC) was created to bring together clinicians, scientists, researchers, and advocates to educate and inform patients and their clinicians and to provide them with options. This book is an important asset in helping the IBC-IC achieve this mission.

Massimo Cristofanilli, MD, FACP

Introduction

This book highlights the progress that has been made in the past few years in diagnosing and treating IBC. It also includes stories from patients describing how they navigated the medical system, found the right doctors, adjusted to treatment protocols, and ultimately, emerged with renewed energy and purpose. For women who have IBC or who might one day be diagnosed with IBC and for the primary care doctors and specialists who might encounter patients with IBC, this book is for you.

When Patti Bradfield and Dr. Massimo Cristofanilli published the book *Nobody Is Listening: Stories of Inflammatory Breast Cancer* In 2014, the outlook for patients diagnosed with IBC was not promising. Patients were often misdiagnosed, and few treatments were available. While misdiagnosis is still a problem, more doctors today are aware of the unusual presentation of IBC, and more patients are being cured.

This book, a sequel to the 2014 book, is written to continue educating doctors and women about IBC and to provide details about recent research, current treatments, and future possibilities that we hope will lead to an even brighter future for women diagnosed with IBC.

Part 1:
Medical Progress in Understanding and Treating IBC

1 IBC Epidemiology

Paul H. Levine, MD, and Carmela Veneroso, MPH

Introduction

Considerable progress has been made in defining the risk factors for developing IBC and discovering what determines long term survival. Eight years ago we[1] noted the obstacles to obtaining appropriate data on this disease, focusing on the lack of a consistent case definition and the relatively small population of patients. Now there is more agreement on identifying IBC patients and there is increasing understanding that IBC should no longer be considered a subcategory of locally advanced breast cancer (LABC). Furthermore, international communication has improved, expanding the patient population available for evaluation. Additionally, the improved correlation of clinical and epidemiological information with laboratory findings has added to the clarification of what IBC is.

Resolving the Case Definition

When IBC was first identified, a unified case definition did not exist. A single case definition is important for both research and diagnosis to ensure that reports by various groups can be applied to all patients with IBC. For example, the important

---

1   Levine et al 2010.

findings (such as effective treatments) emanating from one research group might be overlooked by another research group because the patients are not recognized as IBC patients. On an individual level, physicians might not recognize a patient with IBC because they rarely see an IBC patient and the symptoms do not fit with their preconception of what IBC is. The relative rarity of the disease, the absence of a single case definition, and the fact that it can look more like an infection than cancer are major factors that contribute to misdiagnosis.

Early Case Definitions

The recognition of IBC is attributed to Sir Charles Bell[2] who observed in 1816 that "a purple color on the skin over the tumor accompanied by shooting pains is a very unpropitious beginning."

The term "inflammatory" was introduced by Lee and Tannenbaum[3] who used the term to describe a malignancy in which "as the disease progresses, the skin becomes deep red or reddish purple, and to the touch is brawny and infiltrated. The inflamed area presents a distinct raised periphery after the fashion of erysipelas. The examiner with his eyes closed...can distinguish the sharp contrast between normal and affected tissue."

This clinical definition was the only one used until 1938, when Taylor and Meltzer[4] stated that histological[5] documentation of lymphatic obstruction, which had been suggested earlier by Bryant,[6] provided "pathologic proof" of IBC.

American Joint Committee on Cancer (AJCC) Case Definition

The case definition for the American Joint Committee on Cancer, responsible for developing a uniform staging system

---

2   Bell 1816.
3   Lee and Tannenbaum 1924.
4   Taylor and Meltzer1938.
5   Histological refers to structures visible under a microscope.
6   Bryant T: 1889.

for cancer, has evolved over the years. In its first edition in 1977, AJCC considered IBC to be Stage T4d*[7] but specified it with an asterisk, stating that "inflammatory breast cancer is a clinicopathologic entity...that permeates dermal lymphatics." By 2002, however, the sixth edition stated that "inflammatory carcinoma is a clinicopathologic entity characterized by diffuse erythema and edema[8] (peau d'orange) of the breast, often without an underlying mass. These clinical findings should involve the majority of the breast....It is important to remember that inflammatory carcinoma is primarily a clinical diagnosis. Involvement of the dermal lymphatics alone does not indicate inflammatory carcinoma in the absence of clinical findings." In 2010, the seventh edition[9] broadened the case definition, recognizing IBC to involve less than half the breast. It states that "the term "inflammatory carcinoma" be restricted to cases with typical skin changes involving a third or more of the skin of the breast. While the histologic presence of invasive carcinoma invading dermal lymphatics is supportive of the diagnosis, it is not required, nor is dermal lymphatic invasion without typical clinical findings sufficient for a diagnosis of inflammatory breast cancer."

Surveillance Epidemiology and End Results (SEER) Case Definition

As the AJCC was developing its case definition, the National Cancer Institute (NCI) was developing the Surveillance Epidemiology and End Results (SEER) Program using highly qualified regional population-based cancer registries for epidemiologic studies. In 1973, the 8530 code was assigned which required invasion of the dermal lymphatics with tumor emboli. Clinical inflammation was not considered until 1988,

---

7   T4d* is a clinical stage. T represents topography or tumor size with T4 designating the largest size tumors. The letters a-d signify the extent of tumor invasion with d being specifically to indicate inflammatory breast cancer.

8   Erythema and edema refer to reddening of the skin and swelling caused by excess fluid

9   AJCC- 2010.

when SEER allowed clinical manifestations to be included by linking extent of disease (EOD) codes. In 1988, EOD-E 70 corresponded to the AJCC T4d* designation, i.e., "inflammatory carcinoma, including diffuse (beyond that directly overlying the tumor) dermal lymphatic permeation or infiltration." EOD-S 998 was described as "diffuse, widespread: three quarters or more of the breast; inflammatory breast cancer."[10] Of interest is that SEER required three quarters of the breast, whereas AJCC at that time required only one half or more of the breast.

Over time, as epidemiologic studies developed with SEER co-authors or as consultants,[11] the SEER case definition broadened to allow cases with clinical manifestations involving only one third of the breast.

The French/Tunisian Case Definition

At the same time that IBC was being defined as an important entity in the U.S., French clinicians were developing a different approach to IBC. Denoix at the Institut Gustave Roussy in Paris recognized IBC as an extremely aggressive form of breast cancer and coined the term pousee evolutive (PEV) meaning rapidly progressive breast cancer.[12] He described three phases:

- PEV 3 with clinical involvement covering more than half of the breast was clearly the equivalent of IBC as defined by the American Joint Committee on Cancer (AJCC).
- PEV 2 with clinical signs limited to less than half the breast was considered an earlier manifestation of IBC in France, but was not recognized as IBC in the US although it was definitely of acute onset, rapidly progressing, and with classic clinical signs of IBC.
- PEV 1 with no skin manifestations of IBC but with rapid tumor growth, was identified first by the patient and confirmed by the physician. It had the same poor outcome

---

10   The breast cancer codes begin on page 98 of the SEER coding manual at https://seer.cancer.gov/archive/manuals/historic/EOD_1988.pdf.

11   Levine et al 1985; Chang et al 1998b, Hance et al 2005.

12   Denoix 1977.

as PEV 2 and PEV 3, but it has not been recognized in the US as being related to IBC.

The term PEV 0 came to be used for non-IBC breast cancer, which does not have rapid growth.

The PEV classification has become important because it was used in Tunisia, where IBC affected approximately half of the breast cancer patients seen in the Institut Salah Azaiz, the country's National Cancer Institute[13] and the studies in Tunisia have proven important to help understand the pathogenesis of IBC wherever it exists.

The IBC Registry Case Definition

Because of the challenge of IBC and the need for a uniform case definition, in 2002 Levine, Veneroso, and Zolfaghari developed the IBC Registry (IBCR) and a biospecimen repository with funding from the Department of Defense and the Inflammatory Breast Cancer Research Foundation to "clarify the epidemiology and biology of these tumors."[14] They established a registry of 181 patients from the United States and Canada who had been given the diagnosis of IBC by a clinician and who provided their histories, medical records and tissue blocks for laboratory studies to determine if specific diagnostic markers could be identified that would define the disease.

Since the two primary US organizations that defined IBC had different case definitions when we established our IBC Registry, we classified our patients into the following six categories:

- Cat. 1, displaying redness, warmth, and edema in more than half of the breast with dermal lymphatic invasion
- Cat. 2, displaying redness, warmth, and edema in more than half of the breast with no dermal lymphatic invasion
- Cat. 3, displaying redness, warmth, and edema in less than half of the breast with dermal lymphatic invasion

13   Tabbane et al 1977.
14   Levine et al 2010.

- Cat. 4, displaying redness, warmth, and edema in less than half of the breast with no dermal lymphatic invasion
- Cat. 5, having only dermal lymphatic invasion[15]
- Cat. 6, displaying redness, warmth and edema associated with dermal lymphatic invasion at the site of previously removed non-IBC breast cancer (also called secondary IBC).[16] It is considered to be a result of surgical trauma.[17]

With these categories we collaborated with laboratories who looked for various markers in the specimens of the patients within these categories.[18] The major finding from these studies was that our proposed laboratory markers for IBC were similar among all categories except category 5, thus indicating that the extent of clinical breast involvement and the presence or absence of dermal lymphatic invasion were unimportant in deciding whether the patient had IBC.

Essentially, from the laboratory perspective, the sudden appearance of redness of the breast leading to the detection of cancer cells underneath by biopsy or aspiration indicated that the patient had IBC. Also, several studies have shown that dermal lymphatic invasion alone with no clinical manifestations did not predict an aggressive course with a poor outcome.[19]

Laboratory Studies Using PEV Case Definitions

The early laboratory studies were performed on Tunisian tissue blocks and used PEV case definitions.

Hormone Receptor Studies

The first of our laboratory studies using the classification of IBC patients into subgroups began with our Tunisian study of the

---

15 Called "occult IBC" by Saltzstein, Saltzstein, S. L., Clinically occult inflammatory carcinoma of the breast. *Cancer* 1974, *34*, 382-388.
16 Taylor and Meltzer 1938.
17 Baum 2004, Hashmi 2012.
18 McCarthy et al 2002; Silvera et al 2009, Levine et al 2012; Hoffman et al 2012, Jhaveria et al 2016.
19 Lucas and Perez-Mesa 1978, Amparo et al 2000, Gruber et al 2004.

hormone receptors,[20] which used PEV categories and showed no difference between PEV 1 and PEV 3 but marked differences with PEV 0. One analysis focused on estrogen receptors, as the presence of estrogen receptors is associated with less aggressive breast cancers and signifies an opportunity to use estrogen antagonists such as tamoxifen or aromatase inhibitors in treatment. This study measured the mean level of estrogen receptors and found the mean levels in PEV 1 tumors[21] were similar to PEV 3 tumors[22] and both were significantly lower than the mean level in PEV 0 tumors.[23]

Microvessel Density and Other Markers

The second study using tumors from the same Tunisian cases investigated microvessel density as a marker of angiogenesis, a feature strongly associated with IBC, as well as four other biologic markers, including estrogen receptor status.[24] The study found that greater microvessel density and the estrogen receptor positivity distinguished the PEV 2 and 3 from PEV 0. The study also showed that PEV 1 cases resembled the PEV 2 and 3 cases, but those data were not published. Since PEV 1 is no longer included in epidemiological studies, even in Tunisia,[25] it is unlikely we will see its biological and epidemiological significance demonstrated.

Laboratory Studies Using AJCC and SEER Case Definitions

Recent laboratory studies were performed on tissue blocks from the IBC registry and used AJCC and SEER case definitions.

In 2012[26] we studied several markers of aggressiveness comparing IBC to locally advanced breast cancer (LABC), a form of breast cancer that is usually a neglected tumor and presents

20 Levine et al 1984b.
21 19.0 +/- 6.6.
22 17.9 +/- 6.1
23 30.4 /- 9.2
24 McCarthy et al 2002.
25 Maalej et al 2008.
26 Levine et al 2012.

with a large mass that may resemble IBC but does not have the same tendency to disseminate tumor cells quickly throughout the body. LABC may be treated initially with chemotherapy as is IBC but the rationale is to reduce the size of the tumor allowing easier surgical removal, whereas for IBC the rationale is to eliminate the micro-metastases that may be disseminated before they have a chance to take hold.

In this study of 100 IBC cases from our registry and 107 non-IBC LABC cases seen in a NCI Co-operative program, we divided the IBC cases according to our categories and referred to them as classic IBC (Cats 1 and 2) and atypical IBC (Cats 3 and 4) We looked at the following markers: vascular endothelial growth factor D (VEGF-D), E-cadherin levels, and lymphatic vessel density. We compared the expression of these markers in the classic IBC cases vs LABC cases, and in atypical IBC cases vs LABC cases. There were similarities in the expression of these markers between classic IBC and atypical IBC cases, but significant differences of these markers between the IBC cases and the LABC cases. In looking at the expression of e-cadherin, atypical IBC cases were even more distinct from the LABC cases than were the classic IBC cases. This study concluded that both the AJCC and the SEER case definitions, which currently require clinical symptoms in at least one third of the breast, should be broadened to include patients in categories 3 and 4, where clinical symptoms are found in less than half of the breast.

Etiologic Studies

Considerable information regarding the causes of IBC indicates that the primary contributors are environmental rather than genetic. This section will focus first on population-based data supporting the overall environmental factors that may be contributing and then discuss specific risk factors that would put individuals at higher risk of developing IBC.

Racial/Ethnic Variation

Population-based registries report the incidence of IBC in US breast cancer patients is between 1% and 3%,[27] with variations in the rates largely due to differences in the case definitions used. In the studies of IBC in the US, different ethnic/racial groups also had different incidence rates. All studies showed that Black women have significantly higher rates of IBC than other groups, and some studies showed that Asian and Pacific Islander women had the lowest rates.[28, 29]

Geographical Variation and Time Trends

The notable difference in geographic variation, first suggested by early reports in Tunisia, have been confirmed over time with the development of a population-based registry in Tunisia. Although U.S.-Tunisian disparities are affected by the Tunisians using PEV and the U.S. using IBC, several studies clearly document the higher incidence of IBC in Tunisia.[30, 31] The study authors

---

27 Chang et al 1998b, Wingo et al 2004, Hance et al 2005, Anderson et al 2006.

28 Hance et al 2005, Wingo et al 2004, Goldner et al 2014.

29 Hance et al. found that IBC rates were statistically significantly higher in black women (3.1) than in white women (2.2); Wingo et al. found that Black women had the highest risk (1.6) compared to White women and Asian and Pacific Islander women had the lowest (0.7).In a more recent analysis, Goldner et al found the greatest incidence among black women (3.0), intermediate among white women (2.1) and lowest among Asian women (1.4). Hirko et al,'s study of breast cancer patients from the California, Detroit and New Jersey Surveillance, Epidemiology and End Results (SEER) registries looked at the percentage of Arab Americans who were diagnosed with IBC to investigate a potentially high risk group based on the north African pattern. They identified IBC in only 1.7% of Arab American breast cancer patients compared to 2.91% of American Indian/Alaska patients, 2.3 of Hispanic patients, 2.2% among non-Hispanic Black patients, 1.3% among non-Hispanic Whites and 1.2% among Asians.

30 Maalej et al 1999, Maalej et al 2008, Boussen et al 2010.

31 In the first population-based study which reviewed all breast cancer patients in 1994, 23.2% were classified as PEV 2 or 3. The subsequent study in 2008 evaluated all breast cancer cases in 2004, and the result was similar, 24.3% classified as PEV 2 or 3. In both studies, the more

concluded that IBC was decreasing over time, although the differences in case definition and source of patients makes a precise understanding of the apparent reduction in percentage of IBC cases difficult. Considering the decline in Tunisia contrasting with the steady rise in the incidence of IBC in the United States during the late 1990s,[32] plausible explanations included different patterns of risk factors in the two countries concurrent with the time trends; in Tunisia, socioeconomic conditions have improved while in the United States obesity, one of the most accepted risk factors for IBC, has become rampant.[33] Recent data, however, indicate that the incidence of IBC in the U.S. is decreasing.[34]

Socioeconomic Factors

Descriptions of patterns of IBC suggest that a lower socioeconomic status is a factor in the cause of the disease. In Tunisia, lower socioeconomic status was originally indicated by a rural predominance,[35] and an apparent national decline of IBC occurred with improved socioeconomic conditions.[36] In the United States, Scott et al[37] suggested socioeconomic influences in a study of spatial clustering of county-based IBC rates drawn from the United States Cancer Statistics database. Evidence of spatial clustering was statistically significant, where the average

---

prominent PEV 3 was less frequent than PEV 2, 6.2 and 6.7% compared to 17 and 17.6% respectively. The contrast to Boussen's ISA hospital-based series 1969-1974 (48.7% for PEV 3 and 6.5% for PEV 2) was dramatic. This hospital based study utilized PEV 3/T4D for their case definition of IBC, and although the non-inclusion of PEV-2 cases resulted in fewer cases being evaluated, the overall pattern of disease remained the same with less patients diagnosed with PEV than in earlier years. Interestingly, in a series of 729 cases collected at a university hospital in Tunis 1990-1996 14% of breast cancer cases were reported as PEV 3/T4D in comparison to only 5.7% at ISA, the same hospital that noted 48.7% three decades earlier.

32 Chang et al 1998b, Hance et al 2005, Levine et al 1985.
33 Imes and Burke 2014.
34 Goldner et al 2014.
35 Mourali et al 1980.
36 Boussen et al 2010.
37 Scott 2017.

rates of IBC in the high rate clusters were approximately 12 times the rates in the low rate clusters. High rate clusters, which are less common than low rate clusters,[38] tend to be more urban than rural, have a higher proportion of Blacks, and have a higher percent of the population in poverty. These data were supported by a study using SEER data on the county level[39] which showed that incidence rates for IBC increased as socioeconomic status decreased. In contrast, non-IBC breast cancer has the opposite pattern. Denu et al[40] also noted that IBC patients were more likely to come from areas of higher poverty.[41] In a nested case-control study comparing 617 IBC cases, 1151 LABC cases, 7600 other breast cancer cases, and 93,654 control subjects, all matched by age and year of diagnosis, Schairer et al[42] found a higher level of education was associated with a decreased risk of IBC.

Specific Risk Factors

While most studies of risk factors for breast cancer distinguish between pre-menopausal and post-menopausal breast cancer, in the US the smaller numbers of patients with IBC have not made such separations feasible. The importance of this approach, however, was strongly suggested by the Tunisian studies[43] which described risk factors that are clearly different in pre-menopausal and post-menopausal women. Most dramatic was early age at birth of first child, with 14 of 15 pre-menopausal women in the study who gave birth at the age of 18 or younger being diagnosed with IBC. In post-menopausal women, late menarche was a risk factor as was delay in diagnosis. While rural residence and delay in diagnosis were risk factors in both pre- and post-menopausal women, the relative impact of each risk

38   n=46 for high rate vs n=126 for low rate
39   Schlichting et al 2012.
40   Denu et al 2017.
41   25.6% were at or lower than the 20% poverty level as compared to LABC (21.4%) and non-IBC non-LABC breast cancer (17.4 %, p=0.01).
42   Schairer et al 2013.
43   Mourali et al 1980.

factor was notably different indicating the need to consider the two populations separately in etiologic studies.

Pre-Menopausal Breast Cancer

Hormonal stimulation appears to be the driving force in triggering IBC in younger women. The most important risk factors are obesity, early age at first birth, and prolonged breast feeding.

Obesity: A number of studies have documented obesity as defined by BMI as a major risk factor for pre-menopausal IBC in contrast to non-IBC pre-menopausal breast cancer.[44, 45] Schairer et al. also found that greater mammographic breast density was associated with a statistically significant increased risk of IBC compared to non-IBC breast cancer cases.

Early age at birth of first child: The importance of early age at birth of first child, noted by Mourali et al,[46] was partially confirmed in a subsequent study by Chang et al,[47] who noted that age at birth of first child was lower in the IBC group compared to the non-IBC breast cancer group and the group with other cancers,[48] but the difference was not statistically

---

44 Chang et al 1998a, Schairer et al 2013.

45 Chang et al. found that in sixty-eight 'histologically-confirmed' IBC patients treated at the University of Texas M.D. Anderson Cancer Clinic during the years 1985 to1996, that the highest BMI tertile had a 2.45 statistically significant increased risk for IBC compared to non-IBC. In Schairer et al.'s study of 617 IBC cases, 1151 locally advanced invasive breast cancer (LABC) cases and 7600 of non-inflammatory and non-LABC breast cancer cases from the Breast Cancer Surveillance Consortium (which consists of seven population-based mammography registries), they found that those who were obese (as defined by BMI of greater or equal to 30) had a statistically increased risk of IBC. Their multivariable analyses included pre-menopausal and peri/postmenopausal case subjects together. They found a 3.90 increased risk in pre-menopausal women, 3.70 increased risk in peri/post-menopausal women not currently using hormones, and 2.94 increased risk in in peri/post-menopausal women currently using hormones.

46 Mourali et al 1980.

47 Chang et al 1998a.

48 21.2 in the IBC group compared to 23.0 in the non-IBC breast cancer group and 23.2 in the group with other cancers

significant. This study did not focus on the age group younger than 18, but in a study focusing on the age group that bore their first child before age 20,[49] we noted approximately a 3.2 increased odds of having a higher grade tumor,[50] which is a sign of aggressive breast cancer.

Prolonged breast feeding: A study[51] comparing 49 French IBC patients with 139 non-IBC controls showed a significant effect of prolonged breast feeding in the IBC patients. Women who breast fed 25 or more months[52] were more at risk than those who breast fed 7 to 24 months.[53] As noted by these authors, numerous reports including two recent metanalyses[54] showed that breast feeding was shown to decrease the risk of non-IBC breast cancer proportional to the length of time, thereby indicating another risk factor markedly different in IBC and non-IBC breast cancers.

Post-Menopausal Breast Cancer

Hormonal stimulation is not a factor in triggering IBC in older women. Two risk factors prominent in IBC in Tunisia are delay in diagnosis and late menarche.

Delay in Diagnosis: Although both pre-menopausal and post-menopausal IBC patients had a significantly longer delay in diagnosis than non-IBC breast cancer patients, in post-menopausal patients it is a leading risk factor for IBC. Tabbane et al[55] speculated that in view of the rapid transition observed from PEV 1 and 2 to PEV 3, there may also be a sudden transition from PEV 0 to PEV 1-3. Therefore it is reasonable to assume that the longer a PEV 0 tumor exists untreated, the longer the patient has the risk of developing PEV1-3, or IBC.

---

49 Veneroso et al 2008.
50 OR=3.20; 95% CI=1.20, 8.49
51 Le 2006.
52 OR = 6.7 (2.5-18.3), P=.001 testing for trend
53 OR=2.3 (1.0-5.2)
54 Bernier et al 2000, Collaborative Group on Hormonal Factors in Breast Cancer 2002.
55 Tabbane et al 1977.

The delay in diagnosis could explain why rural women in Tunisia have higher rates of IBC than urban women. In a study of the mean tumor size in the population-based Tunisian Cancer Registry in 2004, Maalej et al[56] found that in 1437 new cases of IBC, tumors seen in public clinics were larger (mean size= 42.5 mm) than those seen in private clinics (mean size= 32.3 mm). The larger tumor size indicates a delay in diagnosis, as the tumor has had more time to grow. Since rural women are more likely than urban women to use public clinics because of their lower socioeconomic status, they are more likely to have larger tumors and therefore higher rates of IBC.

Late menarche: Mourali et al[57] found that late menarche was associated with post-menopausal IBC in Tunisia, even though women in urban Tunisia tend to have menarche at a later age than women in rural Tunisia, and rural residence in Tunisia is shown to be associated with increased risk of IBC.

Genetics

Family history: Overall, studies to date indicate that genetics may have a role in IBC etiology but to no greater extent than non-IBC breast cancer. In a study by Schairer et al,[58] 617 IBC patients, 1151 LABC patients, and 7600 breast cancer patients were compared to 93,654 controls, matched on age and year at diagnosis (which for controls would be a diagnosis of no cancer). In the multivariable rate analyses, they found that the risk ratios of persons with a family history of breast cancer for each breast cancer group did not vary much among the three breast cancer groups[59] but did differ from the controls. The percentage of patients who had a family history of breast cancer was 19.6% for IBC, 18.3% for LABC, and 19.6% for breast cancer, and the percentage for controls was 14.1%.

In another study conducted by Moslehi et al,[60] 141 IBC patients were compared to 178 non-randomized non-IBC

---

56   Maalej et al 2008.
57   Mourali et al 1980.
58   Schairer et al 2013.
59   IBC 1.52 (1.15 to 2.01), LABC 1.40 (1.12 to 1.77), BC 1.38 (1.29 to 1.48)
60   Moslehi et al 2016.

patients (adjusted for age, parity, BMI, regular alcohol use, whether they had ever used oral contraceptives). They found that 17% of the IBC cases had a first-degree breast cancer family history, where as 24.4% of the non-inflammatory breast cancer patients had a family history. They also compared the IBC patients with 465 post-menopausal breast cancer cases from the Hormone Therapy Trials of the Women's Health Initiative (WHI) unselected for family history, and found that 16.9% of the breast cancer patients had a family history, the same percentage as in the IBC patients. They also compared the IBC patients with 9317 healthy controls from the WHI trial with no personal history of breast cancer and found that 12.6% of the healthy controls had a family history. In these several studies, they found that the IBC patients were no more likely than non-IBC breast cancer patients to have a family history of breast cancer, but were more likely than controls to have a family history of breast cancer.

In an analysis of 68 histologically confirmed IBC cases, 143 women age matched and diagnosed with non-IBC breast cancer, and 134 women with cancers other non-breast cancer at M.D. Anderson in the United States, 13% of IBC cases reported a family history of breast cancer versus 8% of the non-IBC breast cancer cases, but this difference was not statistically significant.[61]

Blood Type A: One report indicated a relationship to blood type A in Tunisian women, 43% of women with IBC being A+ compared to 32% of women with non-IBC breast cancer and 33% of a large population of healthy blood donors.[62, 63]In a subsequent independent study, the association with blood type A was confirmed[64] but HLA typing for A, B and DRW antigens revealed no specific IBC-associated antigen.[65] A relationship between blood type A and IBC has not been evaluated in other populations.

---

61 Chang et al 1998a.
62 Mourali et al 1980.
63 Based on the experience of the Tunis Transfusion Center (P=.011)
64 43% vs. 32% in healthy subjects
65 Levine et al 1981.

Local Trauma to the Breast

Observational studies have suggested various triggers to IBC, one significant precipitating agent being local trauma to the breast. Taylor and Meltzer[66] first described two forms of IBC, the primary form where the clinical characteristics are apparent from the outset, and secondary IBC, where the clinical features appear subsequent to treatment for non-IBC breast cancer. The classic rash and pathologic confirmation of dermal lymphatic invasion are typical of secondary IBC. The suggestion that trauma could precipitate aggressive cancer has been noted previously.[67] In our IBC Registry, nine patients had secondary IBC and three additional cases of trauma were reported: seat belt trauma immediately prior to the appearance of IBC in one patient, IBC occurring less than one month after a painful ductogram in a 63-year-old woman with fibrocystic disease, and IBC occurring in a healthy 33-year-old woman shortly after an elective nipple piercing.

Acute Exposures

Time-space cancer clusters, defined as a number of new cases appearing in a short period of time, are always of great interest because they can suggest a specific environmental trigger of the disease in the area of the cluster. Unlike the clustering study described above, time-space clustering can identify a specific agent for the cluster that may not be important in another cluster; the trigger for one could be infectious and for another it could be a toxic spill.[68]

There are three characteristics that are critical to indicate a cancer cluster that is worth investigating for an environmental trigger.

- The cluster should consist of only one type of cancer.
- The cancer should be a rare cancer.

66   Taylor and Meltzer1938.
67   Benish et al 2010, Demicheli et al 2008, Retsky et al 2010.
68   Levine et al 2014.

- The cancer should have a short time period between the causative trigger and the appearance of the cancer (called a latent period).

The last is important because most cancers have a long latent period and the cells divide slowly and at a variable rate so a time-space cluster is not a likely result. IBC fits all of these criteria. It is a relatively rare cancer and has a rapid growth with a short doubling time of cancer cells.

We have reported several clusters of IBC[69] and noted the possible contribution of chemical and infectious triggers. The term "triggering agent" is used because it indicates an environmental agent that has exposed a community but there are apparently other factors, such as genetic susceptibility, that determine which people in the exposed community get the disease.

Chemical exposure: In one IBC cluster we reported[70] there was a confluence of genetics and environmental exposures that could have caused the IBC that developed within a 10-month period in three women who worked in an office of 24 long-term employees. The risk factors identified in the women included office location (a part of the office with poor air and water quality), exposures to herbicides and pesticides, hormone replacement therapy at the time of diagnosis, family history of breast cancer, and obesity. None of the three had all risk factors and conclusions cannot be drawn from three individuals, but each woman had some of the risk factors.

Infectious agents: Some evidence for infection as an environmental triggering agent comes from our study showing that the onset of IBC in two patient populations was less per month in winter months than during the rest of the year.[71, 72]

---

69 Levine et al 2014, Duke et al 2010.
70 Duke et al 2010.
71 Levine et al 2016.
72 n=306, 20.3 for winter months, 27.2 for the rest of the year.

Non-Acute Exposures

Several risk factors have been noted for IBC which were not reported specifically by menopausal status.

Oral contraceptives and alcohol: In the study of heredity and selected environmental factors reported by Moslehi et al,[73] a significant contribution of oral contraceptive use and alcohol consumption (greater than one drink per day) was noted for when IBC patients were compared to two large groups of healthy women (controls in the Women's Health Initiative and controls from a University of Toronto). The use of oral contraceptives was also significantly greater in the IBC cases than in non-IBC breast cancer cases in the Women's Health Initiative. In addition, the oral contraceptive use was slightly (though not significantly) greater in the IBC cases than the non-IBC cases in a George Washington University study.

HMTV virus: Another possible risk factor that has been considered for IBC is a human virus similar to the mouse mammary tumor virus (MMTV), which a group at Mount Sinai Medical Center calls the human mammary tumor virus (HMTV). Support for the presence of this virus comes from at least five different laboratories[74] and studies of human breast milk suggest that as in mice, breast feeding is the usual mode of transmission.[75] The possible association with IBC comes from the observation of a higher prevalence of the mouse-like gp52 antigen in Tunisian breast cancer patients compared to U.S. breast cancer patients[76] and the high prevalence of HMTV-sequences in U.S. IBC patients compared to U.S. non-IBC breast cancer patients.[77] It is not known whether the increased

---

73   Moslehi et al 2016.
74   Ford et al 2003, Pogo et al 2010, Axel et al 1972, Etkind et al 2000, Levine et al 2004.
75   Nartey et al 2014, Johal et al 2011.
76   Levine et al 1984a.
77   The possible association with IBC comes from the observation of a higher prevalence of the mouse-like gp52 antigen in Tunisian breast cancer patients compared to U.S. breast cancer patients(74) and the high prevalence of HMTV-sequences in U.S. IBC patients compared to U.S. non-IBC breast cancer patients.(75). MMTV-related antigen was found in

replication of the suspected virus is a result of more rapid tumor growth or the cause.

Familial aggregation: Other evidence of chronic exposures triggering IBC are suggested by familial aggregation of IBC, which has been reported rarely. A case of familial IBC reported to the IBC Registry that is clearly unrelated to genetics involves a husband and wife with IBC, the husband being diagnosed with IBC 5 years after the onset in his wife.[78]

Survival Studies

Response to Chemotherapy

The barriers to rapid diagnosis and treatment have been shown to exist for both patients and providers,[79] but a prospective cohort study from 155 patients enrolled in the IBC Registry showed that immediate response to neoadjuvant chemotherapy, the standard form of primary treatment for IBC, was the most important determinant for prolonged survival.[80] The patients in this study received combination chemotherapy, usually with three drugs including Adriamycin and cyclophosphamide. Chemotherapy response was significantly associated with observed survival;[81] women not responding to chemotherapy had a significantly higher risk of death compared with women with complete[82] or partial[83] response. These data, confirmatory of a previous clinical trial at MD Anderson,[84] are important as they represent the population of patients seen in private practice outside of clinical trials.

23/33 (70%) Tunisian breast cancers as compared to approximately 35% of U.S breast cancer cases. There was no difference between Tunisian PEV cases (8/12 or 67% positive) and Tunisian non-PEV breast cancer cases (12/17 or 71% positive).

78 P. Levine, personal communication
79 Hashmi et al 2012, Hoffman et al 2012.
80 Hoffman et al 2012.
81 P=0.0030
82 hazard ratio=5.76
83 hazard ratio=3.40
84 Cristofanilli et al 2003.

Speed of Diagnosis

Delay in diagnosis, although not showing as great an effect on survival as response to chemotherapy, did show a trend with a progressive decrease in survival associated with longer delays in diagnosis.[85] The major obstacle to early diagnosis in young women was the resemblance of IBC to acute infection. Common comments from physicians include "breast cancer doesn't hurt" and "you are too young to get breast cancer."[86] The major delays in diagnosis occurred in the time period managed by primary care health care workers, including ob-gyn doctors, with rapid resolution once the patient was referred to a breast specialist. Long term antibiotic use was common with up to five months of multiple antibiotics being used before the diagnosis of cancer was considered.

Socioeconomic Status

Socioeconomics also play an important role in determining outcome. In a study of 7,624 cases of invasive carcinoma identified by cancer registries in seven states, Denu et al[87] observed that in the 170 IBC patients, worse outcomes were seen in patients with Medicaid, patients from urban areas, and patients from areas of higher poverty and lower education. The IBC Registry data noted that factors contributing to delayed diagnosis included lack of medical insurance and attention to other priorities, including co-morbidities that obscured the seriousness of the problem. Denu et al also noted the importance of co-morbidities, which were significantly higher in number and severity than in non-IBC breast cancer patients.

Controlling IBC

Regarding the control of IBC, there are several opportunities for improved detection and treatment.

---

85   Hashmi et al 2012, Hoffman et al 2012.
86   Hashmi and Levine 2017.
87   Denu et al 2017.

Earlier Diagnosis

On the immediate practical level, delay in diagnosis contributes to increased mortality (Hoffman, Hashmi) and earlier diagnosis, primarily achieved by educating physicians and the public, is amenable to intervention.

Regarding physicians, the relative rarity of IBC is a major reason why primary care physicians, including ob-gyn doctors, are unfamiliar with the disease and initially miss the diagnosis. Rapid diagnosis and treatment is the rule once the patients sees a breast specialist,[88] but physicians must be able to recognize IBC, be aware that breast cancer is not always painless, and never think that a patient is too young to have breast cancer.

Educating women to pay attention to breast abnormalities and not be satisfied with unresolved symptoms is also important. We have encountered numerous examples of women diagnosing their problem by searching the web after an unsatisfactory discussion with a primary caregiver. Several other potentially remediable problems are more difficult to solve, such as lack of health insurance and the overwhelming burden of other comorbidities or lifestyle issues that make an apparently minor problem with the breast appear insignificant by comparison.

Treatment Response

There are potential contributions from the laboratory that should be investigated as well. One area of interest is the marked difference in the response of individuals to similar combinations neoadjuvant chemotherapy, which is the standard of care for this disease. Since initial response to treatment is apparently the most important determinant of long term survival (Cristofanilli, Hoffman), an investigation into possible genetic or other determinants of response to treatment should be possible in this era of personalized medicine.

---

88   Hashmi and Levine 2017.

Identifying Markers

Many investigators believe IBC is a unique entity with particular biological properties associated with early metastases, and if this is true, there should be some laboratory markers that show it to be unique. The recent focus on immunotherapy should prompt a search for specific surface antigens that could be the target of this approach. Should such markers be identified, earlier diagnosis and treatment would be an important outcome. Also, at some time in the future it should be possible to know if PEV1 is an early form of IBC. This is an issue of importance in understanding the epidemiology of this disease.

Specifying Risk Factors

The recent findings from several studies indicate that poverty, urban environment, and less education[89] are risk factors for IBC in the U.S. This is in striking contrast to the risk factors for non-IBC breast cancer. IBC patterns in Tunisia show that rural residence is a risk factor for IBC. The common feature in both countries is that urban areas in the US and rural areas in Tunisia have the relatively low income. Income is related to pregnancy patterns because less affluent women often have their first pregnancy at a younger age. While pregnancy is protective against non-IBC breast cancer, a woman who is quite young when her first child is born is at far higher risk of developing IBC. The relative contributions of these various risk factors can be dissected only in analytic studies, such as case-control studies that collect data from individuals rather than populations.

Summary

While IBC continues to be a frightening dangerous malignancy with high morbidity and mortality, the picture has improved dramatically in recent years with improvements in early recognition and treatment. Continued research in various areas, including epidemiology, may not only uncover more

---

89   Scott 2017, Denu 2017, Schairer 2013

opportunities to control IBC but may also uncover factors that make other breast cancers aggressive.

References

AJCC- Edge SB, Byrd DR, Compton CC, Fritz AG, Greene FL, Trotti A, editors. *AJCC Cancer Staging Manual* (7th ed). New York, NY: Springer; 2009.

Amparo RS, Angel CD, Ana LH, Antonio LC, Vicente MS, Carlos FM, Vicente GP. Inflammatory breast carcinoma: pathological or clinical entity? *Breast Cancer Res Treat*, *64*, 269-273; 2000.

Anderson WA, Schairer C, Chen BE, Hance KW, Levine PH. Epidemiology of Inflammatory Breast Cancer (IBC) *Breast Disease* 22: 9-23, 2006.

Axel R, Schlom J, Spiegelman S. Presence in human breast cancer of RNA homologous to mouse mammary tumour virus RNA. *Nature*. 235: 32-36, 1972.

Baum M. Does the act of Surgery provoke activation of "latent metastasis" in early breast cancer? *Breast Cancer Res*, 6:160-161; 2004.

Bell C. *A System of Operative Surgery Founded on the Basis of Anatomy*, Hale and Hosmer: Hartford, CT 1816.

Benish M, Ben-Eliyahu S. Surgery as a double-edged sword: A clinically feasible approach to overcome the metastasis-promoting effects of surgery by blunting stress and prostaglandin responses, *Cancers*, 2: 1929-1951, 2010.

Bernier MO, Plu-Bureau G, Bossard N, Ayzac L, Thalabard JC. Breast feeding and risk of breast cancer: a meta-analysis of published studies. *Hum Reprod* 6:374-86, 2000.

Boussen H, Bouzaine H, Farouk B, Amor G, Mourali N, Monia H, Khaled R, Levine PH. Inflammatory breast Cancer in Tunisia. *Cancer.* 116:2730-2735, 2010.

Bryant T, *Disease of the Breast. Wood Medical and Surgical Monographs IV*, 1889.

Chang S, Buzdar AU, Hursting SD, Inflammatory breast cancer and body mass index, *J Clin Oncol* 16, 3731–3735, 1998a.

Chang S, Parker SL, Pham T, Buzdar AU. Hursting SD. Inflammatory Breast Carcinima Incidence and Survival. *Cancer* 82:2366-2372, 1998b.

Collaborative Group on Hormonal Factors in Breast Cancer. Breast cancer and breastfeeding: collaborative reanalysis of individual data from 47 epidemiological studies in 30 countries, including 50,302 women with breast cancer and 90,973 women without the disease. *Lancet;* 360: 187-95, 2002.

Cristofanilli M, Buzdar AU, Hortobagyi GN. Update on the management of inflammatory breast cancer. *Oncologist*; 8:141-8, 2003.

Demicheli R, Retsky MW, Hrushesky WJ, Baum M, Gukas ID. The effects of surgery on Tumor growth: A century of investigatons. *Ann Oncol* 19: 1821-1828, 2008.

Denoix P. Treatment of malignant breast cancer. Recent Results *Cancer Res*. 92-94, 1977.

Denu RA, Hampton JM, Currey A, Anderon RT, Cress RD, Fleming ST, Lipscomb J, Wu XC, Wilson JF, Trentham-Doetz A. Racial and Socioeconomic Disarities are more Pronounced in Inflammatory Breast Cancer than Other Breast Cancers. *Jl of Cancer Epidemiology* Volume 2017, Article ID 7574946, 2017. doi.org/10.1155/2017/7574946.

Duke TJ, Jahed NC, Veneroso CV, Da Roza R, Johnson O, Hoffman D, Barsky SH, Levine PH. A Cluster of Inflammatory Breast Cancer (IBC) in an Office Setting: Additional Evidence of the Importance of Environmental Factors in IBC Etiology. *Oncology Reports*. 24:1277-1284; 2010.

Etkind P, Du J, Khan A, Pillitteri J, Wiernik PH. Mouse mammary tumor virus-like ENV gene sequences in human breast tumors and in a lymphoma of a breast cancer patient. *Clin Cancer Res*. 2000;6: 1273-1278.

Ford CE, Tran D, Deng Y, Ta VT, Rawlinson WD, Lawson JS. Mouse mammary tumor virus-like gene sequences in breast tumors of Australian and Vietnamese women. *Clin Cancer Res*.;9: 1118-1120, 2003.

Goldner B, Behrendt CE, et al. "Incidence of inflammatory breast cancer in women, 1992-2009, United States." *Ann Surg Oncol* 21(4): 1267-70, 2014.

Gruber G, Ciriolo M, Altermatt HJ, Aebi S, Berclaz G, Greiner RH. Prognosis of dermal lymphatic invasion with or without clinical signs of inflammatory breast cancer. *Int J Cancer*, *109*, 144-148, 2004.

Hance K, Anderson W, Devesa S, Young HA, Levine PH. Trends in Inflammatory Breast Cancer Incidence and Survival: The Surveillance, Epidemiology, and End Results Program at the National Cancer Institute. *Jl Nat Cancer Inst* 97: 966-975, 2005.

Hashmi S, Zolfaghari L, Levine PH. Does Secondary Inflammatory Breast Cancer Represent Post-Surgical Metastatic Disease? *Cancers.* 4: 156-164; 2012. doi: 10.3390/cancers401056;

Hashmi S and Levine PH. Barriers to Early Diagnosis of Inflammatory Breast Cancer. *Insights Breast Cancer* 1:2.2, 2017.

Hoffman HJ, Levine PH, Paul L, Khan A, Ajmera K, Schendfeld J. Initial response to chemotherapy, not delay in diagnosis, predicts overall survival in inflammatory breast cancer. *Am J of Clin Oncol.* 2012; doi: 10.1097/COC.0b013e318271b34b.

Imes CC and Burke LE. The Obesity Epidemic: The United States as a Cautionary Tale for the Rest of the World. *Curr Epidemiol Rep.* June 1(2) 82-88, 2014. doi: 10.1007/s40471-014-0012-6.

Jhaveria K, Teplinsky E, Silvera S, Valeta-Magara A, Arju R, Giashuddin R, , Sarfraz Y, Alexander M, Darvishian F, Levine PH, Hashmi S, Zolfaghari L, Hoffman HJ, Singh B, Goldberg J, Hochman T, Formenti S, Esteva FJ, Moran MS Schneider RJ. Hyperactivated mTOR and JAK2/STAT3 Pathways: Molecular Drivers and Potential Therapeutic Targets of Inflammatory and Invasive Ductal Breast Cancers After Neoadjuvant Chemotherapy. *Clinical Breast Cancer.* Apr;16(2):113-22.e1., 2016 doi: 10.1016/j.clbc.2015.11.006. Epub 2015 Dec 1.

Johal H, Ford C, Glenn W, Heads J, Lawson J, Rawlinson W. Mouse mammary tumor like virus sequences in breast milk from healthy lactating women. *Breast Cancer Res Treat.* 2011 Aug;129(1):149-55. doi: 10.1007/s10549-011-1421-6. Epub 2011 Mar 2.

Le MG, Arriagada R, Bahi J, et al. Are risk factors for breast similar in women with inflammatory breast cancer and in those with non-inflammatory breast cancer? *Breast* 15: 355-362. 2006.

Lee B. and Tannenbaum N. "Inflammatory carcinoma of the breast: a report of twenty-eight cases from the breast clinic of Memorial Hospital." *Surg Gynecol Obstet* 39: 580-595. 1924.

Levine PH, Mourali N, Tabbane F, Loon J, Terasaki P, Tsang P, Bekesi JG. Studies on the role of cellular immunity and genetics in the etiology of rapidly progressing breast cancer in Tunisia. *Int J Cancer* 27:611-615, 1981.

Levine PH, Mesa-Tejada R, Keydar I, Tabbane F, Spiegelman S, Mourali N. Increased incidence of mouse mammary tumor virus-related antigen in Tunisian patients with breast cancer. *Int J Cancer* 33:305-308, 1984a.

Levine PH, Tabbane F, Muenz LR, Kamaraju LS, Das S, Polivy S, Belhassen S, Scholl SM, Bekesi G, Mourali N. Hormone receptors in rapidly progressing breast cancer. *Cancer* 54(12):3012-3016, 1984b.

Levine PH, Steinhorn SC, Ries LG, Aron JL. Inflammatory breast cancer: the experience of the Surveillance, Epidemiology and End Results (SEER) Program. *J Natl Cancer Inst* 74:291-297, 1985.

Levine PH, Pogo BG, Klouj A, et al. Increasing evidence for a human breast carcinoma virus with geographic differences. *Cancer.*101: 721-726. 2004.

Levine PH, Zolfaghari L, Young H, Hafi M, Cannon T, Ganesan C, Veneroso C, Brem R, Sherman M. What Is Inflammatory Breast Cancer? Revisiting the Case Definition. *Cancers. 2:* 143-152; 2010.

Levine PH, Portera CC, Hoffman HH, Yang SX, Takikita M, Duong QN, Hewitt SM, Swain SM. Evaluation of Lymphangiogenic Factors, Vascular Endothelial Growth Factor D and E-Cadherin in Distinguishing Inflammatory from Locally Advanced Breast Cancer. *Clinical Breast Cancer*. 12: 231-239; 2012.

Levine PH, Hashmi S, Minaei AA, Veneroso C. Inflammatory Breast Cancer Clusters: A Hypothesis. *World J Clin Oncol.* 5(3): 539-545; 2014. http://dx.doi.org/10.5306/wjco.v5.i3.539.

Levine PH, Liu Y, Veneroso C, Hashmi S, Cristofanilli M. Seasonal Variation in Inflammatory Breast Cancer. *Int J I* 4(1) , 17-21, 2016.

Lucas FV, Perez-Mesa C. Inflammatory carcinoma of the breast. *Cancer, 41,* 1595-1605; 1978.

Maalej M, Frikha H, Ben Salem S, Daoud J, Bouaouina N, Ben Abdellah M, Ben Romdahane K, Breast Cancer in Tunisia: a clinical and epidemiological study. *Bull Cancer*: 86:302-306, 1999.

Maalej M, Hentati D, Messai T, Kochbati L, El May A, Mrad K, Ben Romdahane K, Ben Abdellah M, Zouari B. Breast cancer in Tunisia in

2004:a comparative clinical and epidemiological study. *Electronic Jl. Of Oncology Bull Cancer* 95: E5-9, 2008.

McCarthy N, Linnoila I, Merino M, Paik S, Parr A, Levine P, Hewitt S, Swain S. Inflammatory Breast Cancer is Associated with an Increased Microvessel Density Compared with Non-Inflammatory Breast Cancer. *Clinical Cancer Research* 8: 3857-3862, 2002.

Moslehi R, Freedman F, Zeinomar N, Veneroso C, Levine PH. Importance of hereditary and selected environmental risk factors in the etiology of inflammatory breast cancer: a case-comparison study. *BMC Cancer* 16:334-343, 2016.

Mourali, N., Muenz, L.R., Tabbane, F., Belhassen, S., Bahi, J., and Levine, P.H. Epidemiologic features of rapidly progressing breast cancer in Tunisia. *Cancer* 46 (12) :2741-2746, 1980.

Nartey T, Moran H, Marin T, Arcaro KF, Anderton DL, Etkind P, HollandJF, Melena SM, Pogo BG-T. Human Mammary Tumor Virus (HMTV) sequences in human Milk. *Infect Agent Cancer*.9: 20. 2014. Published online 2014 Jun 17. doi: 10.1186/1750-9378-9-20

Pogo BG, Holland JF, Levine PH. Human mammary tumor virus in inflammatory breast cancer. *Cancer*.116: 2741-2744, 2010.

Retsky M, Demicheli R, Hrushesky WJ, Baum M, Gukas ID. Surgery triggers outgrowth of latent distant disease in nreast cancer: An inconvenient truth? *Cancers* 2: 305-337, 2010.

Schairer C, Li Y, Frawley P, Graubard BI, Wellman RD, Buist DS, Kerlikowske K, Onega TL, Anderson WF, Miglioretti DL: Risk factors for inflammatory breast cancer and other invasive breast cancers. *J Natl Cancer Inst*, 105(18):1373-1384, 2013.

Schlichting JA, Soliman AS, Schairer C, Schottefeld D, Merajver SD. Inflammatory and noninflammatory breast cancer survival by socioeconomic position in the Surveillance, Epidemiology and End Results data base, 1990-2008. *Breast Cancer Research and Treatment*, 134: 1257-1268, 2012. doi:10.1007/s10549-012-2133-2.

Scott L, Mobley LR, Il'yasova. Geospatial Analysis of Inflammatory Breast Cancer and Associated Community Characteristics in the United States. *Int J Environ Res Public Health* April 11, 2017. doi: 10.3390/ijerph10404.

Silvera D, Arju R, Darvishian F, Levine PH, Zolfaghari L, Holdberg J, Hochman T, Formenti SC, Schneider RJ. Essential role for elF4Gl overexpression in the pathogenesis of inflammatory breast cancer. *Nature Cell Biology* 11:903-908, 2009. doi: 10.1038/ncb1900.

Tabbane F, Muenz L, Jaziri M, Cammoun M, Belhassen S, et al. Clinical and prognostic features of a rapidly progressing breast cancer in Tunisia. *Cancer*.40: 376-382.11. 1977.

Taylor and Meltzer, Inflammatory carcinoma of the breast. *Am J Cancer*. 33:33-49, 1938.

Veneroso C, Siegel R, Levine PH. Early age at first childbirth associated with advanced tumor grade in breast cancer. *Cancer Detect Prev* 32: 215-223, 2008.

Wingo PA, Jamison PM, Young JL, Gargiullo P. Population-based statistics for women diagnosed with inflammatory breast cancer (United States). *Cancer Causes and Control* 15: 321-328, 2004.

2 Molecular Basis of IBC

Sangjucta Barkataki, PhD, Madhura Joglekar-Javadekar, PhD, and Kenneth L. van Golen, PhD

Background

Inflammatory Breast Cancer (IBC) is considered the most aggressive form of epithelial breast cancer.[90] IBC is characterized by its rapid onset progression and being diagnosed as an advanced tumor. Although the incidence of IBC is estimated to be 1-5 percent of breast cancer patients annually in the United States, however it is thought to account for nearly 10 percent of breast cancer deaths.[91] Overall survival of IBC patients is significantly less than other breast cancer patients whether or not metastases are evident at the time of diagnosis.[92] Younger women across all ethnicities with an average age of approximately 55 years are especially affected by IBC.[93] The term "inflammatory" is misleading and it comes from the appearance of the breast. IBC patients present with several skin changes such as erythema (reddening of the skin), edema (swelling

---

90 Woodward 2015.
91 van Golen, K.L. and Cristofanilli, M. 2013.
92 Woodward 2015. van Golen, K.L. and Cristofanilli, M. 2013. Dawood, S. and Valero V. 2012.
93 Woodward 2015. van Golen, K.L. and Cristofanilli, M. 2013. Dawood, S. and Valero V. 2012.

with warmth to the touch) and a skin texture that resembles the skin of an orange (peau d'orange).[94] All of these symptoms resemble an infection. It is estimated that 90 percent of patients are misdiagnosed and are treated extensively with antibiotics.[95] Because the cancer progresses so rapidly, time spent treating with antibiotics may result in a decreased chance of survival for the patient.[96] There is also a form of IBC known as secondary IBC. Primary IBC is the appearance of a rapidly growing breast lump and the skin manifestations noted above. Secondary IBC occurs after treatment of a more slow growing breast cancer with no skin changes and is manifest by redness and an apparent rash at the site of previous surgery.[97] Typically, primary and secondary IBC are distinguished by a short history with the rapid appearance of symptoms which could include pain or itching.[98] This chapter will focus on primary IBC.

IBC often presents without a lump; the tumor cells are in the breast tissue in sheets or cords of cells. A classic characteristic of IBC is infiltration of tumor cells in the dermal lymphatic vessels of the skin overlying the breast. IBC cells form clusters of tumor cells called emboli in the dermal lymphatic vessels. IBC tumor emboli have the ability to spread throughout the body.[99] Because of this, about 1/3 of patients have clinically detectable metastases at the time of diagnosis,[100] but it is likely that non-apparent micrometastases are present early in the disease and appear clinically a year or so after diagnosis.

The current consensus in the field is that IBC is not only unique in its presentation from other forms of breast cancer, but it is also molecularly different.[101] A unique 75 gene signature profile that is closely associated with IBC was identified by a

---

94 Woodward 2015.
95 van Golen, K.L. and Cristofanilli, M. 2013.
96 Hashmi, S. and Levine, P.H. 2017.
97 Hashmi, S. and Levine, P.H. 2017.
98 Dawood, S. and Valero V. 2012.
99 Woodward 2015. Kleer, C.G. et al. 2000. Fouad, T.M. et al.2015.
100 Woodward 2015. Kleer, C.G. et al. 2000. Fouad, T.M. et al.2015.
101 Woodward 2015. Kleer, C.G. et al. 2000. Fouad, T.M. et al.2015.

large collaborative study performed by several groups in the Inflammatory Breast Cancer International Consortium (IBC-IC).[102]

A History of IBC Research

Since its identification and classification by Lee and Tannenbaum in 1924, IBC has remained a misunderstood and underrepresented form of breast cancer in terms of research focus.[103] Its classification as a distinct entity has been argued for the better part of a half-century. A detailed review of the literature over the span of 80 years starting from 1924 suggests that the infrequency of IBC coupled with its misdiagnosis, typically as 'mastitis', are the reasons why IBC has been largely ignored until recently. Early studies included single or a few incidental IBC samples in comparison with conventional breast cancers. Early studies assumed IBC to be comparable to other breast cancers and they attempted to relate IBC to conventional breast cancers.

The Presence of Receptors on IBC Tumor Cells

Early studies focused on markers on the surface of breast cancer cells that reflect biologic features of the cancer. These markers are called receptors and indicate individual features of each tumor, including some that may be susceptible to treatment which interrupts the biology of the cancer growth. The receptor status of IBC was examined. The percentage of estrogen receptor positive (ER+) and progesterone receptor positive (PR+) cases were lower in IBC compared to stage-matched locally advanced breast cancers (LABC; ER+, 44 percent versus 64 percent; PR+, 30 percent versus 51 percent, respectively).[104] In another early study, analysis for expression of ER and PR, HER-2, the epidermal growth factor receptor (EGFR) was also measured.[105] The study demonstrated that of the IBC samples analyzed, less than 40 percent were slightly ER, PR positive,

---

102 Van Laere, S.J. et al.2013.
103 Lee, B. J. and Tannenbaum, N.E. 1924.
104 Paradiso, A. et al. 1989.
105 Charpin, C. et al. 1992.

while 58 percent were EGFR positive and 60 percent expressed HER-2. IBC tumors can also lack expression of ER/PR and HER-2 and are referred to as triple negative (TN). As in conventional breast cancers, ER/PR positive tumors carry a better prognosis, while TN tumors have the worst prognosis.

The Importance of Receptors in Treatment

ER positive tumors tend to be good candidates for aromatase inhibitors and tamoxifen, as these drugs modulate estrogen. Similarly, HER2+ tumors are often treated with Herceptin, which is a specialized antibody used to target the HER2 receptor on the surface of the breast cancer cell. Herceptin is often used in combination with other chemotherapies. Unfortunately, tumors lacking ER/PR and HER-2 are considered to be triple negative and lack these receptors as targets for additional therapies. The EGFR can be targeted in any tumors expressing it, including triple negative breast cancers.

To this point IBC research was effectively studying the role of these diagnostic and prognostic factors on overall survival of IBC patients, similar to non-IBC studies. Although important, none of these studies addressed the invasive nature of IBC. In regards to the unique clinical presentation of IBC compared to non-IBC, nearly nothing was known about the contrasting features between these two-breast cancer types with respect to their genetic basis. Our laboratory was one of the first few labs that started looking at the genetic dissimilarities within these two cancer groups.

The Importance of Genes in Understanding the Aggressive Characteristics of IBC

All cells in the body contain the same genes. However, the characteristics and behavior of a cell are determined by which genes are active and being "expressed". Gene expression is the process by which a cell takes information from a gene and synthesizes a functional gene product, such as a protein. It is the functional protein that effects a cells behavior. For example, both skin and liver cells contain the same genes, however the expression of genes in each cell type is different, allowing different functional proteins to be produced leading to the specialized characteristics of each cell type. In 1999, Drs. van Golen and Merajver published a study specifically focused on IBC and testing the hypothesis that that the disease was metastatic almost upon its inception. Using a modified technique they compared genes which are expressed from the newly-established SUM149 triple negative IBC cell line, normal human mammary cells (HMECs) and lymphocytes from the patient that the SUM149 was derived.[106] Seventeen differentially expressed genes were identified and confirmed using another technique. Some genes were found to be expressed in IBC cells and not in normal breast cells, while other genes were not expressed in IBC cells compared to the normal cells. To determine which genes were absolutely unique to IBC, expression of each of the identified genes was measured in IBC patient samples and tumor stage-matched non-IBC specimens. Expression of two genes were found to be specifically and significantly altered in IBC patient samples: a novel gene that was cloned and called Lost in Inflammatory Breast Cancer (LIBC) and RhoC GTPase. Results of this study were further confirmed by Vermeulen and colleagues five years later using tissue microarray analysis.[107]

Expression of LIBC was lost in 80 percent of inflammatory tumors and 21 percent of non-inflammatory tumors. Over time LIBC has been renamed as IGF binding protein-related protein 9 (IGFBP-rP9), CCN9 and most recently Wnt1-inducible secreted protein 3 (WISP3). WISP3 is thought to be a tumor suppressor gene in IBC.[108]

How IBC Cells Move

RhoC GTPase, is a molecule that is involved in making cells move. Normally, RhoC is only expressed by white blood cells involved in moving toward infections. However, RhoC GTPase was overexpressed in 90 percent of inflammatory tumors,

---

106 van Golen, K.L. et al. 1999.
107 Van den Eynden, G.G. et al. 2004.
108 Kleer, C.G. et al. 2002.

whereas only 38 percent of non-inflammatory tumors.[109] To study the role of RhoC GTPase in contributing towards IBC invasion, we expressed the RhoC gene in normal human mammary epithelial cells (HMECs). The HMEC-RhoC GTPase cells were found to be highly motile and invasive. When injected into the mammary fat pad of mice, the cells grew tumors. These studies were the first to show that RhoC GTPase transfected mammary epithelial cells carry the ability to generate cellular effects that strikingly resemble the *in vivo* IBC phenotype.[110] We still do not know how or why RhoC GTPase is expressed in IBC; however, we have determined how it is activated, leading to invasion. Akt1 is a protein known for helping cells survive. However in IBC it has another function: it leads to the activation of RhoC GTPase through phosphorylation. Activation of Akt1 in IBC, but not any other cell type, leads to RhoC phosphorylation and invasion.[111] Loss of caveolin-1 expression, is associated with non-IBC tumor progression, however in IBC this protein is overexpressed.[112] Caveolin-1 is a protein involved in organizing other proteins at the cell membrane so that they can effectively "talk to" one another. In IBC cells, overexpression of caveolin-1 is required for the activation of Akt1 leading to activation of RhoC and invasion.[113]

How IBC Emboli May be Formed and Hold Together

Coupled with research demonstrating unique expression patterns of molecular markers known to be altered in non-IBC, the identification of RhoC GTPase gave insights into the unique molecular profile associated with IBC metastasis. E-cadherin is a molecule on the surface of cells that normally holds epithelial cells, such as those that line the milk ducts of the breast, together. Loss of E-cadherin expression is typically associated with progression of a number of cancers including breast

---

109 van Golen, K.L. et al. 1999.
110 Joglekar, M. and van Golen, K.L. 2012.
111 Lehman, H.L. et al. 2012.
112 Van Den Eynden, G.G. et al. 2006.
113 Joglekar M. et al. 2015.

cancer. However, E-cadherin is overexpressed in IBC.[114] The overexpression of E-cadherin may help to explain how IBC cells can form tumor emboli.

Recent Progress in IBC Research

Over the past decade, IBC research has made significant progress giving further clues into the drivers of the unique phenotype of the disease and providing potential new therapeutic targets. Identification of the protein Alk, which is involved in lung cancer cell growth, has been identified as potential therapeutic target for IBC.[115] Similarly, a study demonstrated IBC patients who had taken statins were shown to have significantly improved progression-free survival.[116] In turn these findings led to a line of investigation demonstrating that IBC uses cholesterol differently than normal breast or other types of breast cancer.[117] Use of the cholesterol-lowering statin, Simvastatin, sensitizes IBC tumors to radiation, improving IBC outcomes.[118]

The Development of New Ways to Study IBC in the Laboratory

Techniques for growing and studying IBC in the laboratory has also improved significantly; our laboratory developed a novel system to culture IBC emboli in the lab. To do this we reproduced the physical and mechanical properties of the dermal lymphatic system. In this culture system, only tumor cells that are able to invade the lymphatic system such as IBC (but not non-inflammatory breast cancer) or melanoma, readily form tumor emboli in the laboratory.

114 Kleer, C.G. et al. 2001. Tomlinson, J.S. et al. 2001.
115 Tuma, R.S. et al. 2011.
116 Brewer et al. 2013.
117 Wolfe, A.R. 2015
118 Lacerda 2014.

Understanding the Biology of IBC Using a New Model System

The emboli culture system has improved the study of IBC by placing the tumor cells in an environment that stimulates the formation of biologically-relevant emboli. Arora et. al. identified high levels of anti-apoptotic proteins in IBC tumor emboli by adapting the culture system to high-throughput analysis.[119] The simplicity of the model lends itself both to conventional molecular and phenotype analysis as well as a high-throughput approach. The growth of IBC cells as tumor emboli allows for a better representation of how the cells would behave in the body. An overview of this was presented at the 2018 IBC-IC meeting in Madrid, Spain. Several laboratories have utilized this 3D emboli culture system to study different biological aspects of IBC emboli biology with success. Effects of the tumor microenvironment on IBC tumor stem cells, specifically hybrid epithelial/mesenchymal cells, were effectively studied using this model system.[120] The role of molecules involved in inflammation, such as transforming growth factor beta (TGFβ) and interleukin-6 (IL-6), were shown to drive signaling in tumor stem cells.

The Role of Stem Cells and IBC

A major research effort has focused on the origins of IBC. Recent evidence suggests a large cancer stem cell population in IBC tumors and dermal lymphatic emboli.[121] Stem cells have the ability to renew themselves almost indefinitely, and have the ability to give rise to cells that are more specialized. Tumor cells isolated from models of human IBC have been found to express both proteins seen in embryo cells and also what had been described for breast cancer stem cells.[122] Further, 74 percent of human IBC samples express cancer stem cell markers, which is significantly higher than the 44 percent of non-IBC cells.[123]

---

119 Arora et al. 2017.
120 Bocci et al. 2019 .
121 van Golen, C.M. and van Golen, K.L. 2012.
122 van Golen, C.M. and van Golen, K.L. 2012.
123 van Golen, C.M. and van Golen, K.L. 2012.

Our laboratory used IBC patient samples compared with non-IBC patient samples and identified overexpression of the platelet-derived growth factor receptor alpha (PDGFRA). PDGFRA is a receptor for a growth factor that normally is involved in wound healing and formation of new blood vessels. PDGFRA is often seen to be abnormally expressed in cancer like gastrointestinal stromal tumors and glioblastoma. We demonstrated that activity of PDGFRA was shown to be associated with shorter metastasis-free survival in IBC patients. Using IBC cell lines grown in the emboli culture system, activity of PDGFRA was inhibited by the small molecule inhibitor Crenolanib (CP-868-596). Crenolanib treatment interfered with IBC cell growth and emboli formation in culture and tumor growth in mice, reducing tumor size by 3-fold.

Taking on New Challenges in IBC Research

One problem that affects IBC patients is the formation of skin metastases after they have completed treatment. Skin metastases reduce the quality of life of the patient and also can reduce life-expectancy. Although significantly different diseases, IBC and melanoma share a number of similarities both in presentation and progression. Both cancers spread via dermal lymphatics, form intralymphatic emboli and have a propensity to form skin metastases.[124] Melanoma can also present as "inflammatory melanoma", which resembles IBC in appearance.[125] Thus, new leads for studying cutaneous metastasis can be gathered from the melanoma literature. Studies demonstrate a role for the inflammatory molecule TGFβin the formation of melanoma skin metastasis.[126] TGFβ promotes tumor cell invasion and its expression can be induced in the stroma by radiation treatment.[127] Recent studies describe low expression of the growth factor TGFβ in IBC patients, which

---

124 Woodward 2015. Leiter, U. et al. 2004. Rose, A.E. et al. 2011.
125 Haupt, H.M. et al. 1984.
126 Perrot, C.Y. et al. 2013. Schmid, P. et al. 1995.
127 Barcellos-Hoff, M.H. 1993. Cichon, Magdalena A. et al. 2011. Ehrhart, E.J. et al. 1997. Giampieri, S. et al. 2009. Gotzmann, J. et al. 2004. Mukai, M. et al. 2006.

may promote cohesive invasion of IBC cells.[128] TGFβ normally controls functions like cell growth and survival. Stimulation of IBC cells with TGFβ causes altered tumor cell behavior such as stimulating single cell invasion. Study have shown that cells from the emboli are able to invade in clusters via RhoC GTPase-dependent amoeboid movement and this invasion by clusters of IBC cells is disrupted by exposure to TGFβ.[129]

Concluding Remarks

Since 1999, IBC research has made great strides in understanding the overall biology of the disease. This chapter was an overview of a small portion of the studies that have been conducted and published on IBC. The global conclusion of these studies is that IBC is a molecularly distinct disease in comparison to non-IBC. As investigators continue to tease out the molecular basis of IBC, new improved therapies will be developed.

---

128 van Golen, K.L. and Cristofanilli, M. 2013. Lehman, H.L. et al. 2012.
129 Lehman, H.L. et al. 2012.

References

Arora et al. *Oncotarget,* 2017 Apr 18;8(16):25848-25863. doi: 10.18632/oncotarget.15667.

Barcellos-Hoff, M.H., Radiation-induced Transforming Growth Factor β and Subsequent Extracellular Matrix Reorganization in Murine Mammary Gland. *Cancer Res*, 1993. **53**(17): p. 3880-3886.

Bocci et al. PNAS January 2, 2019 116 (1) 148-157; published ahead of print December 26, 2018. doi.org/10.1073/pnas.1815345116.

Brewer et al. *Br. J. Cancer* 2013, 109(2) 318-324.

Charpin, C., et al. Inflammatory breast carcinoma: an immunohistochemical study using monoclonal anti-pHER-2/neu, pS2, cathepsin, ER and PR. *Anticancer Res*, 1992. **12**(3): p. 591-7.

Cichon, Magdalena A., Evette S. Radisky, and Derek C. Radisky, Identifying the Stroma as a Critical Player in Radiation-Induced Mammary Tumor Development. *Cancer Cell*, 2011. **19**(5): p. 571-572.

Dawood, S. and V. Valero, Clinical Aspects of Inflammatory Breast Cancer: Diagnosis, Criteria, Controversy, in *Inflammatory Breast Cancer: An Update*, N.T. Ueno and M. Cristofanilli, Editors. 2012, Springer: New York, N.Y. p. 11-20.

Ehrhart, E.J., et al. Latent transforming growth factor beta1 activation in situ: quantitative and functional evidence after low dose gamma-irradiation. *FASEB*, 1997. **11**: p. 991-1002.

Fouad, T.M., et al. Overall survival differences between patients with inflammatory and noninflammatory breast cancer presenting with distant metastasis at diagnosis. *Breast cancer research and treatment*, 2015. **152**(2): p. 407-416.

Giampieri, S., et al. Localized and reversible TGFbeta signalling switches breast cancer cells from cohesive to single cell motility. *Nat Cell Biol*, 2009. **11**(11): p. 1287-96.

Gotzmann, J., et al. Molecular aspects of epithelial cell plasticity: implications for local tumor invasion and metastasis. *Mutat.Res.*, 2004. **566**(1): p. 9-20.

Hashmi S, Levine PH. Barriers to Early Diagnosis of Inflammatory Breast Cancer. *Insights of Breast Cancer* 2017; 1:2.1.

Haupt, H.M., A.F. Hood, and M.H. Cohen, Inflammatory melanoma. *J Am Acad Dermatol*, 1984. **10**(1): p. 52-5.

Joglekar M. et al. Caveolin-1 Mediates Inflammatory Breast Cancer Cell Invasion via the Akt1 Pathway and RhoC GTPase. *J Cell Biochem* 2015; 118(5): 923-33.

Joglekar, M. and K.L. van Golen, Molecules That Drive the Invasion and Metastasis of Inflammatory Breast Cancer, in *Inflammatory Breast Cancer: An Update*, N.T.C. Ueno, M., Editor. 2012, Springer: New York, NY USA. p. 161-184.

Kleer, C.G. et al. *Oncogene* 2002 May 9;21(20):3172-80., doi: 10.1038/sj.onc.1205462.

Kleer, C.G. et al. Persistent E-cadherin expression in inflammatory breast cancer. *Mod Pathol*. 2001; 14(5): 458-64.

Kleer, C.G., et al. Molecular biology of breast cancer metastasis. Inflammatory breast cancer: clinical syndrome and molecular determinants. *Breast Cancer Res*, 2000. **2**(6): p. 423-429.

Lacerda *Stem Cells Transl Med* 2014, 3(7) 849-856.

Lee, B. J. and Tannenbaum, N.E. Inflammatory carcinoma of the breast: a report of twenty-eight cases from the breast clinic of Memorial Hospital. *Surg Gynecol Obstet*, 1924. **39**: p. 580-595.

Lehman, H.L. et al. Regulation of inflammatory breast cancer cell invasion through Akt1/PKBα phosphorylation of RhoC GTPase. *Mol Cancer Res*. 2012 10(10): 1306-18.

Lehman, H.L., et al. Modeling and characterization of inflammatory breast cancer emboli grown in vitro. *Int J Cancer*, 2012.

Leiter, U., et al. The natural course of cutaneous melanoma. *Journal of Surgical Oncology*, 2004. **86**(4): p. 172-178.

Mukai, M., et al. RhoC is essential for TGF-beta1-induced invasive capacity of rat ascites hepatoma cells. *Biochem Biophys Res Commun*, 2006. **346**(1): p. 74-82.

Paradiso, A., et al. Cell kinetics and hormonal receptor status in inflammatory breast cancer. Comparison with locally advanced disease. *Cancer*, 1989. **109**: p. 1922-1927.

Perrot, C.Y., D. Javelaud, and A. Mauviel, Insights into the transforming growth factor beta signaling pathway in cutaneous melanoma. *Ann Dermatol*, 2013. **25**(2): p. 135-144.

Rose, A.E., P.J. Christos, and F. Darvishian, Clinical Relevance of detection of lymphovascular invasion of primary melanoma using endothelial markers D2-40 and CD34. *The American Journal of Surgical Pathology*, 2011. **35**(10): p. 1441-1448.

Schmid, P., P. Itin, and T. Rufli, In situ analysis of transforming growth factor-βs (TGF-β1, TGF-β2, TGF-β3and TGF-3 type II receptor expression in malignant melanoma. *Carcinogenesis*, 1995. **16**(7): p. 1499-1503.

Tomlinson, J.S. et al. An intact overexpressed E-cadherin/alpha,beta-catenin axis characterizes the lymphovascular emboli of inflammatory breast carcinoma. *Cancer Res*. 2001; 61(13): 5231-41.

Tuma, R.S., et al. The Alk gene is amplified in most inflammatory breast cancers. *J Nat Cancer Inst* 2011; 104(2): 87-88.

Van Den Eynden, G.G. et al. *Overexpression of caveolin-1 and -2 in cell lines and in human samples of inflammatory breast cancer.* Breast Cancer Res Treat 2006 95(6): 219-28.

Van den Eynden, G.G. et al. Validation of a tissue microarray to study differential protein expression in inflammatory and non-inflammatory breast cancer. *Breast cancer Res Treat* 2004 85(1): 13-22.

van Golen, C.M. and K.L. van Golen, Inflammatory Breast Cancer Stem Cells: Contributors to Aggressiveness, Metastatic Spread and Dormancy. *Molecular Biomarkers and Diagnosis*, 2012. **S-8**: p. 1-4.

van Golen, K.L. and M. Cristofanilli, The Third International Inflammatory Breast Cancer Meeting. *Breast Cancer Res*, 2013. **15**: p. 318-321.

van Golen, K.L. et al. A novel putative low-affinity insulin-like growth factor-binding protein, LIBC (lost in inflammatory breast cancer), and RhoC GTPase correlate with the inflammatory breast cancer phenotype. *Clin Cancer Res* 1999; 5(9): 2511-2519.

Van Laere, S.J., et al. Uncovering the molecular secrets of Inflammatory Breast Cancer biology: An integrated analysis of three distinct Affymetrix gene expression data sets. *Clinical Cancer Research*, 2013.

Wolfe AR *Int J Radiat Oncol Biol Phys* 2015, 91(5) 1072-80.

Woodward, W.A., Inflammatory breast cancer: unique biological and therapeutic considerations. *The Lancet Oncology*, 2015. **16**(15): p. e568-e576.

3 Treatment

Jennifer M. Rosenbluth, MD, PhD, and Beth A. Overmoyer, MD

Introduction

Inflammatory Breast Cancer (IBC) is an aggressive type of breast cancer that is treated with multiple categories of sequential therapy: drugs that go throughout the body to kill cancer cells, surgery to remove the breast and axillary lymph nodes, and radiation to the local chest wall region.[130] In this chapter we will discuss therapy and therapeutic advances both for IBC that is localized (present in the breast and regional lymph nodes but not in distant parts of the body) and for IBC that has metastasized (spread to distant parts of the body). Although IBC has been associated with worse outcomes, major treatment advances have been developed that are leading to better outcomes for patients than ever before.

Trimodality Therapy for Localized Disease

Treatment of IBC involves multiple disciplines of oncology, and a patient should meet with a medical oncologist, radiation oncologist, and surgical oncologist for the treatment of their disease. At the time of diagnosis, IBC involves the entire breast, skin of the breast, and axillary lymph nodes, so that surgery

---

130 Woodward, W. A. et al. 2017.

is contraindicated for the first line of treatment. Therefore, the initial therapy will involve the use of systemic drugs that target and/or kill cancer cells first. This is followed by surgical procedures (complete mastectomy and axillary lymph node dissection), and then by radiation therapy to the chest wall and regional lymph nodes (axillary, supraclavicular, internal mammary). This is known as "trimodality therapy" and it is associated with improved survival rates in patients with IBC. Although this approach unfortunately remains underutilized, a greater adoption of this approach is one important means by which we are achieving improved outcomes in IBC.[131]

Timing of Drug-Based Therapy

Neoadjuvant Therapy

Many IBC patients are surprised to find that they are being treated with drugs first, before other therapies such as surgery or radiation. When these drugs, such as chemotherapy, are given before surgery it is called neoadjuvant therapy. Neoadjuvant therapy is the cornerstone of treatment for localized inflammatory breast cancer.[132] This is due to a fundamental property of IBC: the cancer cells have gained the ability to invade the blood and lymphatic vessels which can lead to distant spread of tumor cells, even if those cells are below the level of detection. Lymphatic vessels are natural channels in our body that help fluids circulate throughout our tissues and our body. The presence of the IBC cells in the lymphatic vessels of the skin is manifest by redness, swelling, and puckering of the skin of the breast making it look similar to an orange peel (peau d'orange).[133] This property is indicative of the need for upfront therapy to decrease the overall burden of disease. This kills the IBC and allows the breast and lymph nodes to be resected surgically.

131 Rueth, N. M. et al. 2014.
132 Overmoyer, B. A. 2010.
133 Lucas, F. V. & Perez-Mesa, 1978, Cserni, G., Charafe-Jauffret, E. & van Diest, P. J. 2018.

There are additional reasons to give drug-based therapy before surgery in IBC. These include the way that the breast cancer cells are arranged in the tissue of the breast in IBC. Typically, one considers a breast cancer to be a single lump in the breast, but many cases of IBC present without a palpable lump. Instead, the tumor's cells can be loosely infiltrative throughout the tissue of the breast.[134] In other words, they can be scattered throughout a larger region that is harder to define. In addition, they are more likely to spread to regional lymph nodes behind the breast, sternum, and in the axilla that may be harder to treat with surgery. For these reasons, using a therapy that goes to all of these different places, such as chemotherapy, can be helpful to do upfront.

Drug-based therapy is also able to kill cancer cells that have escaped the breast and regional lymph nodes. These cells, which are too small to detect, have spread outside the breast through the lymphatics and through the blood vessels to distant sites in the body. We call this micrometastatic disease. Eradicating micrometastatic disease is essential in order to cure breast cancer, and this can only occur using therapies that disseminate throughout the entire body, such as chemotherapy.

Finally, by receiving drug-based therapy upfront, one can assess the response of the tumor to that therapy. If the patient has already had a mastectomy, there are no visible skin changes and there is no radiographic mass to measure and see if the chemotherapy is working. In contrast, the response to therapy when given before surgery can be assessed by physical exam, radiology (e.g. mammogram, ultrasound, PET-CT, or MRI), and, at the time of surgery, by a pathologist who will look for scar tissue or other signs that tumor cells have been effectively killed by the drugs.

Adjuvant Therapy

In many cases, additional drug-based therapy is given after surgery. This is called adjuvant therapy. The decision on whether and what type of adjuvant therapy to offer patients

---

134 Cserni, G., Charafe-Jauffret, E. & van Diest, P. J. 2018.

has become increasingly complex as more therapies are being developed and as we gain more knowledge about the benefits of extended therapy for certain patients at high-risk of developing metastatic disease. Even in patients with an excellent response to neoadjuvant therapy, some treatment can often be beneficial after surgery with the goal of eradicating remaining micrometastatic disease. In some cases there may be no detectable invasive breast cancer cells in the breast or axillary lymph nodes removed at the time of surgery; this is called a pathologic complete response (pCR).[135] Patients achieving a pCR to neoadjuvant therapy may be able to avoid some adjuvant drug-based therapy, a process we now term "de-escalation of therapy".

The timing and sequence of therapies often differ between IBC and non-IBC patients, and understanding this difference is another means by which outcomes can be improved for IBC patients.

Systemic Therapy Choices

Classes of drugs that are given prior to surgery can include chemotherapy and anti-HER2 therapy, with endocrine therapy administered after surgery; all of these agents are considered systemic therapy because they travel throughout the body to kill cancer cells. The choice of therapy used depends in part on the specific subtype of breast cancer, however all subtypes of IBC are initially treated with chemotherapy. Subtypes of breast cancer are described the same way for IBC and non-IBC. They can be defined by the presence or absence of three markers known as receptors: estrogen receptor (ER), progesterone receptor (PR) and HER2. The two hormonal receptors (ER and PR) are used by normal breast cells to grow at the appropriate time, such as during puberty. But breast cancers sometimes increase these receptors to very high levels, or use other means to activate them, allowing the breast cancer cells to grow in an uncontrolled manner. HER2 is another cellular receptor that primarily supports the heart, but it is activated to stimulate

---

135 Nakhlis, F. et al. 2017.

cancer growth in approximately 40% of IBC compared with 15-20% of non-IBC.[136]

HER2 Positive IBC

HER2 positive breast cancer presents a different target for breast cancer therapy: HER2, which can be blocked to inhibit breast cancer growth and survival. There are a growing number of drugs that target the HER2 receptor. These include antibodies such as trastuzumab (Herceptin) and pertuzumab (Perjeta), which are given in combination with chemotherapy prior to surgery, as well as after surgery. Newer therapies that target HER2 include antibody-drug conjugates and small molecule inhibitors. T-DM1 is an antibody-drug conjugate that links the anti-HER2 antibody trastuzumab directly to a potent molecule of chemotherapy (DM1), in effect bringing the chemotherapy directly to the tumor. Recently, a second antibody-drug conjugate, trastuzumab deruxtecan, has become available to treat HER2 positive breast cancer. Small molecule inhibitors of HER2 include lapatinib as well as neratinib and tucatinib. These newer therapies are currently used for treatment of recurrent or metastatic HER2-positive breast cancer, including IBC, as well as in the adjuvant setting after surgery.

Neoadjuvant Therapy in HER2 Positive IBC

Our ability to target HER2 positive breast cancers, which are more common in IBC than non-IBC, has been a major advance for this type of cancer. As a result, we are seeing more cures for HER2 positive IBC, and the list of drugs that we can use to target HER2 is expanding, which improves our ability to treat this disease in the metastatic setting. Anti-HER2 therapies enhance the efficacy of chemotherapy and are given concurrently with chemotherapy prior to surgery to treat IBC. Standard regimens include THP-AC (paclitaxel/trastuzumab/pertuzumab) followed by doxorubicin/cyclophosphamide; THP is typically given first in order to provide upfront anti-HER2 therapy), or for some patients TCHP (docetaxel/carboplatin/

136 Parton, M. et al. 2004, Cakar, B. et al. 2018, Kertmen, N. et al. 2015.

trastuzumab/pertuzumab). This approach was developed in the context of neoadjuvant clinical trials such as NOAH, which in turn was supported by studies of trastuzumab in combination with chemotherapy in the adjuvant setting.[137] NOAH compared chemotherapy plus trastuzumab (117 patients) to chemotherapy alone (118 patients) for patients with HER2 positive locally advanced or inflammatory breast cancer. The addition of trastuzumab to chemotherapy markedly improved patient outcomes.[138] Subsequent studies that included limited numbers of patients with IBC, NeoSphere and TRYPHAENA, supported the addition of pertuzumab to trastuzumab and chemotherapy in these regimens, as compared to trastuzumab alone.[139]

Adjuvant Therapy in HER2 Positive IBC

The majority of data supporting these recommendations for the systemic treatment of IBC are extrapolated from clinical trials that involve few, if any, patients with IBC, but are designed to improve the outcomes of breast cancer patients in general. The Katherine trial is one such example,[140] and it supports an approach to adjuvant therapy that is tailored to the response of the tumor to neoadjuvant therapy. If a pCR is achieved after neoadjuvant therapy (such as THP-AC), then HER2-based adjuvant therapy should consist of trastuzumab and pertuzumab to complete a total of one year of therapy. However, if there is residual cancer at the time of surgery and pCR is not achieved, then adjuvant therapy should consist of T-DM1 for approximately one year of therapy. These HER2-targeted therapies should be given in conjunction with post-mastectomy radiation therapy, and in the case of hormone receptor-positive disease, in conjunction with endocrine therapy.

It remains an open question whether or not T-DM1 should be given in the adjuvant setting to all patients with inflammatory breast cancer, regardless of whether or not they achieved a pCR, because of the increased risk of disease recurrence with IBC.

137 Perez, E. A. et al. 2011.
138 Gianni, L. et al. 2010.
139 Gianni, L. et al. 2016, Schneeweiss, A. et al. 2013.
140 von Minckwitz, G. et al. 2019.

Additional research in this area is needed. In addition, in HER2+ breast cancer improved outcomes were seen when neratinib, as compared to placebo, was given for one year after the completion of trastuzumab-based adjuvant therapy.[141] Whether or not there is a benefit in patients who received pertuzumab or T-DM1 is not clear. In addition, benefit from neratinib was generally limited to patients who had breast cancer that was both HER2+ and ER+, likely because these two receptors can interact or crosstalk with each other, leading to improved outcomes when both receptors are inhibited in the adjuvant setting.[142]

Triple Negative IBC

For the triple-negative subtype of IBC, the cornerstone of therapy remains chemotherapy since triple negative disease has no known therapeutic target. However, there are a number of clinical trials exploring investigational agents that can be added to chemotherapy. Some examples of these studies are described in greater detail below. Outside of a clinical trial, the standard preoperative chemotherapy regimens include an anthracycline and a taxane. An example of standard therapy is dose-dense doxorubicin and cyclophosphamide (AC) for four cycles followed by paclitaxel given either dose-dense (every two weeks) or weekly for 12 weeks.[143] The role of additional platinum (i.e., carboplatin) is still unclear.[144]

In the adjuvant setting, patients who have residual cancer found at the time of surgery (i.e. do not achieve a pCR) can be offered the oral chemotherapy agent capecitabine, based on the results of the CREATE-X trial.[145]

Hormone Receptor Positive IBC

Fortunately, we have means of targeting the hormone receptors ER and PR using drugs classified as endocrine therapy, such as

141 Martin, M. et al. 2017.
142 Sudhan, D. R. et al. 2019.
143 Woodward, W. A. et al. 2017.
144 Wang, D., Feng, J. & Xu, B. A 2019.
145 Zujewski, J. A. & Rubinstein, L. 2017.

tamoxifen, letrozole, anastrazole, fulvestrant, and exemestane, that all block the activity of ER either directly or by reducing estrogen levels. These agents are used after breast surgery and are often taken for years. For example, in ER/PR positive IBC, chemotherapy is given before surgery, and endocrine therapy may involve pills that are given after surgery and taken daily for ten years.

This is particularly true following the advent of more recent studies which highlight the importance of endocrine therapy for patients at increased risk of recurrence or metastasis. These include studies that show that the duration of endocrine therapy should be increased from five years to ten years for patients at high risk for breast cancer recurrence, such as those with IBC,[146] and studies that show that additional therapy to suppress the ovaries can be added to make endocrine therapy even more effective for certain high risk premenopausal women, again such as those with IBC.[147] IBC is, by definition, a high-risk form of breast cancer, therefore adjuvant therapy that targets high risk individuals should be utilized for patients with IBC. Additional therapies that add targeting agents to standard adjuvant endocrine therapy, such as CDK 4/6 inhibitors (abemaciclib, palbociclib, or ribociclib) may also benefit those patients with hormone receptor positive IBC, although conclusive studies are still pending (ongoing studies: https://clinicaltrials.gov/ct2/show/NCT02513394, https://clinicaltrials.gov/ct2/show/NCT03155997, and https://clinicaltrials.gov/ct2/show/NCT03701334).

Supportive Therapy

Finally, patients are often anxious about chemotherapy because of a perception of intractable nausea or other severe side effects. However, not only has our armamentarium of systemic therapy agents improved, but our ability to manage the side effects of systemic therapy has also improved with time. These include medications to control nausea, to treat diarrhea or

146 Gray, R. & Group, E. B. C. T. C. 2018, Burstein, H. J. et al. 2019.
147 Regan, M. M., Fleming, G. F., Walley, B., Francis, P. A. & Pagani, O. 2019, Francis, P. A., Regan, M. M. & Fleming, G. F. 2015, Francis, P. A. et al. 2015, Pagani, O. et al. 2014.

constipation, and to manage hot flashes and night sweats that can be associated with endocrine therapy.

Assessment of Response

Response to therapy is assessed at every visit by physical examination. Prior to surgery, response is indicated by a decrease in redness of the skin of the breast, decrease in the size of palpable masses in the breast or the lymph nodes, and/or decrease in swelling of the breast. Often, there is improvement in pain or other symptoms from the cancer as well.

Multiple radiographic techniques can also be used to assess response to therapy in the neoadjuvant setting. These include mammogram and ultrasound, which are standard assessments for breast masses and lymph node metastases. These techniques are often not as specific as breast MRI in demonstrating disease response to neoadjuvant therapy. Breast MRI is very useful in IBC as it can reveal a thickening of the tissues of the breast, and non-mass-like enhancement, which describes a radiographic finding in which there is no breast mass but still abnormal signal on imaging that may be of concern. Skin thickening and lymph node enlargement is also demonstrated by MRI imaging. These are all findings that can be associated with IBC and should improve with systemic therapy. Often, the clinical examination is sufficient to determine disease response to treatment; however, breast imaging as described can confirm this finding or, in the case of poor responses to treatment, support changing systemic therapy rather than proceeding to surgery.

There is growing evidence for a role for PET-CT in assessing IBC disease burden at baseline, and in some cases it may be useful for assessing disease response.[148] The vast majority of IBC will give a detectable signal on PET-CT. As a result, PET-CT can sometimes identify cancer in locations where it was not previously detectable by conventional imaging such as CT or bone scan.[149] It can also be useful for subsequent radiation therapy mapping, for example by highlighting IBC in regional

148 Groheux, D. et al. 2013, Jacene, H. A. et al. 2018.
149 Groheux, D. et al. 2013, Jacene, H.A. et al. 2020.

lymph nodes that should be irradiated but were not detected by other means of breast imaging or CT.[150]

If physical examination findings as well as radiographic findings suggest a good response to neoadjuvant therapy, surgery will typically be recommended as the next step. If an inadequate response to therapy is suspected, additional neoadjuvant therapy should be given to achieve the maximal disease response and enable surgical removal of the breast and axillary lymph nodes which contain minimal, if any, IBC.

Local/Regional Therapies

In IBC, the standard-of-care for surgical management is a complete mastectomy, accompanied by a complete axillary lymph node dissection, i.e., removal of level 1 and 2 axillary lymph nodes (modified radical mastectomy). There are a number of studies that support improved outcomes with a modified radical mastectomy in IBC, as compared to breast-conserving therapy (lumpectomy combined with radiation therapy).[151] This includes evidence of an improvement in survival when mastectomy is performed in IBC.[152] Breast conservation remains investigational for IBC, even in the setting of a complete clinical response.

In addition, in other subtypes of breast cancer, sentinel lymph node biopsies may be utilized instead of axillary lymph node dissection, but this is not recommended in IBC. The sentinel lymph node(s) are the first lymph nodes that drain the lymphatic fluid of the breast, and they can be identified intraoperatively by injecting a dye or radioactive material into the breast and tracing its path. However, there is evidence the lymphatic drainage system is altered in IBC due to the presence of the clumps of tumor cells. This results in higher false-negative rates and lower identification rates for sentinel lymph node biopsies, making sentinel lymph node sampling investigational in IBC.[153]

---

150 Walker, G. V. et al. 2012, Jacene, H.A. et al. 2020.
151 Nakhlis, F. et al. 2017, Rosso, K. J. et al. 2017, Hieken, T. J. et al. 2018.
152 Muzaffar, M., Johnson, H. M., Vohra, N. A., Liles, D. & Wong, J. H. 2018.
153 Stearns, V. et al. 2002, DeSnyder, S. M. et al. 2018.

Because rates of recurrence of IBC in the chest wall and regional lymph nodes can be high even after surgery, post-mastectomy radiation is recommended. The purpose of radiation is to kill any dormant IBC cells within the lymphatics of the skin and draining lymph node regions. In addition, in some practices the dose of radiation therapy is changed based upon unique considerations for IBC.[154] A standard radiation approach for IBC includes treatment of the chest wall with a bolus, nodal fields (axillary, supraclavicular and internal mammary), and a boost to the mastectomy incision.[155] Use of drugs to enhance the effectiveness of radiation therapy, called radiosensitizers, is an active area of research and is described in greater detail in the clinical trials section below.

Thus, therapies that prevent local recurrence, which can ultimately lead to distant recurrence, are critical to improving outcomes for IBC patients.

Metastatic IBC

In the setting of metastasis, IBC is treated in a similar manner to non-IBC with a few exceptions. In specific circumstances, evidence suggests a role for local-regional therapy for preventing complications from progressive cancer in the breast and chest wall.[156] In addition, due to a propensity for metastasis to the brain, there is emerging evidence that screening brain MRI may be beneficial in patients with Stage IV IBC at the time of disease progression.[157] Clinical trials can also be an option for patients with metastatic IBC.

Clinical Trials

Clinical trials have become an important part of breast cancer care. These are research studies and participation is entirely voluntary. In some instances, patients choose to participate in trials because they gain access to investigational treatments or

---

154 Woodward, W. A. 2014.
155 Bristol, I. J. et al. 2008, Warren, L. E. et al. 2015a.
156 Warren, L. E. et al. 2015a, Akay, C. L. et al. 2014.
157 Warren, L. E. et al. 2015b.

novel therapeutic approaches. For example, there is growing evidence that therapy that utilizes a patient's own immune system to kill cancer cells may be of particular interest in IBC, but this requires further research, including through clinical trials. Unfortunately, the majority of clinical trials either exclude patients with IBC or the total proportional enrollment from IBC is <1%. This means that there are very few dedicated clinical trials specifically for IBC, and the majority of the standard of care recommendations for the treatment of IBC are extrapolated from predominately non-IBC studies. Here, we highlight a few additional examples of clinical trials that are specific to IBC.

In triple-negative IBC, there is evidence that the cancer cells exhibit some properties similar to cancer stem cells, and these cells can be inhibited by blocking a specific molecular pathway called the JAK-STAT pathway. An ongoing clinical trial evaluates the small molecule JAK1/2 inhibitor ruxolitinib given in combination with chemotherapy in the neoadjuvant setting for newly diagnosed triple-negative IBC (ongoing, https://clinicaltrials.gov/ct2/show/study/NCT02876302).

There is also evidence for another active signaling pathway in tripe-negative IBC: the EGFR pathway. There is recent evidence that EGFR inhibitors such as panitumumab may be efficacious in combination with chemotherapy, again specifically in the neoadjuvant setting in triple-negative IBC[158] (ongoing, https://clinicaltrials.gov/ct2/show/study/NCT01036087).

Additional methods of killing the cancer stem cells that may mediate resistance are being investigated in clinical trials, such as in a Phase II clinical trial of the chemotherapy agent eribulin followed by doxorubicin/cyclophosphamide for HER2-negative IBC (ongoing, https://clinicaltrials.gov/ct2/show/NCT02623972).

As mentioned above, given the presence of infiltrating immune cells in IBC, multiple studies have focused on whether these immune cells promote IBC growth and spread.[159] It remains an open question whether or not drugs that activate the

158 Matsuda, N. et al. 2018.
159 Allen, S. G. et al. 2016, Reddy, J. P. et al. 2018, Valeta-Magara, A. et al. 2019, Wolfe, A. R. et al. 2016, Bertucci, F. et al. 2015, Reddy, S. M. et al. 2019.

immune system to kill cancer cells (immunotherapy) would be particularly effective in IBC. A Phase II clinical trial is investigating the addition of one immunotherapy agent (nivolumab) given in combination with standard chemotherapy for IBC (ongoing, https://clinicaltrials.gov/ct2/show/NCT03742986).

Some drugs can enhance the effectiveness of radiation therapy and are called radiosensitizers, and these are also an active area of research. For example, there is currently an ongoing phase II randomized trial assessing the benefits of the PARP inhibitor olaparib as a radiosensitizer in IBC (ongoing, https://clinicaltrials.gov/ct2/show/study/NCT03598257), based on a promising pilot trial for a similar agent in this disease.[160]

The above clinical trials, open at the time of writing of this chapter, demonstrate that efforts to improve therapy in IBC are an active area of research. Clinical trials are entirely voluntary and are a research effort, but some patients choose to participate in trials because they provide them with the opportunity to be treated with investigational therapies, often in addition to standard therapy rather than replacing it. The list of available clinical trials is constantly changing, but patients with IBC should consider discussing clinical trial options with their treating oncologist.

Improvement in Outcomes in IBC

As a result of better recognition of the disease and advances in therapy, there have been improvements in outcomes for patients with IBC over time. An analysis of patients with Stage III IBC in the Surveillance, Epidemiology and End Results (SEER) Registry was performed for patients diagnosed within four time periods covering two decades. Two-year breast cancer-specific survival rates increased with time as follows: 62% from 1990-1995, 67% from 1996-2000, 72% from 2001-2005, and 76% from 2006-2010.[161]

A separate retrospective analysis of locally advanced breast cancer patients (defined based on staging criteria as having

160 Jagsi, R. et al. 2018.
161 Dawood, S. et al.2014.

"T4" disease), including patients with IBC, was performed using an institutional breast cancer registry from 1990-2014. In this cohort, T4 disease had the largest improvements in disease-free survival over time of any breast cancer subtype.[162] In addition, analysis of patients treated at one center identified 114 patients with inflammatory breast cancer who had received trimodality therapy. Although longer follow-up is needed, improved locoregional control was seen, with only four patients with local regional recurrence in this cohort.[163] These data suggest that improvements in and greater adoption of trimodality therapy can improve outcomes for IBC patients, and that further progress in this regard has the potential to lead to even greater improvements in the future.

Summary

IBC is an aggressive disease, and as a result curative treatment is complicated and utilizes multiple modalities of therapy: neoadjuvant anti-cancer drugs (chemotherapy, HER2 directed therapy), surgery, radiation, and adjuvant endocrine therapy. However, improvements in therapeutic agents and in treatment approaches are leading to improved outcomes for IBC patients. In addition, there is ongoing active and important research which will continue to improve therapy for this disease in the years to come.

162 Malmgren, J. A., Atwood, M. K. & Kaplan, H. G. 2017.
163 Rosso, K. J. et al. 2017.

References

Akay, C. L. *et al.* Primary tumor resection as a component of multimodality treatment may improve local control and survival in patients with stage IV inflammatory breast cancer. *Cancer* **120**, 1319-1328, doi:10.1002/cncr.28550 (2014).

Allen, S. G. *et al.* Macrophages Enhance Migration in Inflammatory Breast Cancer Cells via RhoC GTPase Signaling. *Sci Rep* **6**, 39190, doi:10.1038/srep39190 (2016).

Bertucci, F. *et al.* PDL1 expression in inflammatory breast cancer is frequent and predicts for the pathological response to chemotherapy. *Oncotarget* **6**, 13506-13519, doi:10.18632/oncotarget.3642 (2015).

Bristol, I. J. *et al.* Locoregional treatment outcomes after multimodality management of inflammatory breast cancer. *Int J Radiat Oncol Biol Phys* **72**, 474-484, doi:10.1016/j.ijrobp.2008.01.039 (2008).

Burstein, H. J. *et al.* Adjuvant Endocrine Therapy for Women With Hormone Receptor-Positive Breast Cancer: ASCO Clinical Practice Guideline Focused Update. *J Clin Oncol* **37**, 423-438, doi:10.1200/JCO.18.01160 (2019).

Cakar, B. *et al.* The Impact of Subtype Distribution in Inflammatory Breast Cancer Outcome. *Eur J Breast Health* **14**, 211-217, doi:10.5152/ejbh.2018.4170 (2018).

Cserni, G., Charafe-Jauffret, E. & van Diest, P. J. Inflammatory breast cancer: The pathologists' perspective. *Eur J Surg Oncol* **44**, 1128-1134, doi:10.1016/j.ejso.2018.04.001 (2018).

Dawood, S. *et al.* Survival of women with inflammatory breast cancer: a large population-based study. *Ann Oncol* **25**, 1143-1151, doi:10.1093/annonc/mdu121 (2014).

DeSnyder, S. M. *et al.* Prospective Feasibility Trial of Sentinel Lymph Node Biopsy in the Setting of Inflammatory Breast Cancer. *Clin Breast Cancer* **18**, e73-e77, doi:10.1016/j.clbc.2017.06.014 (2018).

Francis, P. A. *et al.* Adjuvant ovarian suppression in premenopausal breast cancer. *N Engl J Med* **372**, 436-446, doi:10.1056/NEJMoa1412379 (2015).

Francis, P. A., Regan, M. M. & Fleming, G. F. Adjuvant ovarian suppression in premenopausal breast cancer. *N Engl J Med* **372**, 1673, doi:10.1056/NEJMc1502618 (2015).

Gianni, L. *et al.* 5-year analysis of neoadjuvant pertuzumab and trastuzumab in patients with locally advanced, inflammatory, or early-stage HER2-positive breast cancer (NeoSphere): a multicentre, open-label, phase 2 randomised trial. *Lancet Oncol* **17**, 791-800, doi:10.1016/S1470-2045(16)00163-7 (2016).

Gianni, L. *et al.* Neoadjuvant chemotherapy with trastuzumab followed by adjuvant trastuzumab versus neoadjuvant chemotherapy alone, in patients with HER2-positive locally advanced breast cancer (the NOAH trial): a randomised controlled superiority trial with a parallel HER2-negative cohort. *Lancet* **375**, 377-384, doi:10.1016/S0140-6736(09)61964-4 (2010).

Gray, R. & Group, E. B. C. T. C. in *2018 San Antonio Breast Cancer Symposium.* Abstract nr GS3-03 (*Cancer Res*).

Groheux, D. *et al.* 18F-FDG PET/CT in staging patients with locally advanced or inflammatory breast cancer: comparison to conventional staging. *J Nucl Med* **54**, 5-11, doi:10.2967/jnumed.112.106864 (2013).

Hieken, T. J. *et al.* Influence of Biologic Subtype of Inflammatory Breast Cancer on Response to Neoadjuvant Therapy and Cancer Outcomes. *Clin Breast Cancer* **18**, e501-e506, doi:10.1016/j.clbc.2017.10.003 (2018).

Jacene, H. A. *et al.* Metabolic Characterization of Inflammatory Breast Cancer With Baseline FDG-PET/CT: Relationship With Pathologic Response After Neoadjuvant Chemotherapy, Receptor Status, and Tumor Grade. *Clin Breast Cancer*, doi:10.1016/j.clbc.2018.11.010 (2018).

Jagsi, R. *et al.* Concurrent Veliparib With Chest Wall and Nodal Radiotherapy in Patients With Inflammatory or Locoregionally Recurrent Breast Cancer: The TBCRC 024 Phase I Multicenter Study. *J Clin Oncol* **36**, 1317-1322, doi:10.1200/JCO.2017.77.2665 (2018).

Kertmen, N. *et al.* Molecular subtypes in patients with inflammatory breast cancer; a single center experience. *J BUON* **20**, 35-39 (2015).

Lucas, F. V. & Perez-Mesa, C. Inflammatory carcinoma of the breast. *Cancer* **41**, 1595-1605 (1978).

Malmgren, J. A., Atwood, M. K. & Kaplan, H. G. in *2017 San Antonio Breast Cancer Symposium.* (ed AACR) (Cancer Research).

Martin, M. *et al.* Neratinib after trastuzumab-based adjuvant therapy in HER2-positive breast cancer (ExteNET): 5-year analysis of a randomised, double-blind, placebo-controlled, phase 3 trial. *Lancet Oncol* **18**, 1688-1700, doi:10.1016/S1470-2045(17)30717-9 (2017).

Matsuda, N. *et al.* Safety and Efficacy of Panitumumab Plus Neoadjuvant Chemotherapy in Patients With Primary HER2-Negative Inflammatory Breast Cancer. *JAMA Oncol*, doi:10.1001/jamaoncol.2018.1436 (2018).

Muzaffar, M., Johnson, H. M., Vohra, N. A., Liles, D. & Wong, J. H. The Impact of Locoregional Therapy in Nonmetastatic Inflammatory Breast Cancer: A Population-Based Study. *Int J Breast Cancer* **2018**, 6438635, doi:10.1155/2018/6438635 (2018).

Nakhlis, F. *et al.* The Impact of Residual Disease After Preoperative Systemic Therapy on Clinical Outcomes in Patients with Inflammatory Breast Cancer. *Ann Surg Oncol* **24**, 2563-2569, doi:10.1245/s10434-017-5903-6 (2017).

Overmoyer, B. A. Inflammatory breast cancer: novel preoperative therapies. *Clin Breast Cancer* **10**, 27-32, doi:10.3816/CBC.2010.n.003 (2010).

Pagani, O. *et al.* Adjuvant exemestane with ovarian suppression in premenopausal breast cancer. *N Engl J Med* **371**, 107-118, doi:10.1056/NEJMoa1404037 (2014).

Parton, M. *et al.* High incidence of HER-2 positivity in inflammatory breast cancer. *Breast* **13**, 97-103, doi:10.1016/j.breast.2003.08.004 (2004).

Perez, E. A. *et al.* Four-year follow-up of trastuzumab plus adjuvant chemotherapy for operable human epidermal growth factor receptor 2-positive breast cancer: joint analysis of data from NCCTG N9831 and NSABP B-31. *J Clin Oncol* **29**, 3366-3373, doi:10.1200/JCO.2011.35.0868 (2011).

Reddy, J. P. *et al.* Mammary stem cell and macrophage markers are enriched in normal tissue adjacent to inflammatory breast cancer. *Breast Cancer Res Treat*, doi:10.1007/s10549-018-4835-6 (2018).

Reddy, S. M. *et al.* Poor Response to Neoadjuvant Chemotherapy Correlates with Mast Cell Infiltration in Inflammatory Breast Cancer. *Cancer Immunol Res*, doi:10.1158/2326-6066.CIR-18-0619 (2019).

Regan, M. M., Fleming, G. F., Walley, B., Francis, P. A. & Pagani, O. Adjuvant Systemic Treatment of Premenopausal Women With Hormone Receptor-Positive Early Breast Cancer: Lights and Shadows. *J Clin Oncol* **37**, 862-866, doi:10.1200/JCO.18.02433 (2019).

Rosso, K. J. *et al.* Improved Locoregional Control in a Contemporary Cohort of Nonmetastatic Inflammatory Breast Cancer Patients Undergoing Surgery. *Ann Surg Oncol* **24**, 2981-2988, doi:10.1245/s10434-017-5952-x (2017).

Rueth, N. M. *et al.* Underuse of trimodality treatment affects survival for patients with inflammatory breast cancer: an analysis of treatment and survival trends from the National Cancer Database. *Journal of clinical oncology : official journal of the American Society of Clinical Oncology* **32**, 2018-2024, doi:10.1200/JCO.2014.55.1978 (2014).

Schneeweiss, A. *et al.* Pertuzumab plus trastuzumab in combination with standard neoadjuvant anthracycline-containing and anthracycline-free chemotherapy regimens in patients with HER2-positive early breast cancer: a randomized phase II cardiac safety study (TRYPHAENA). *Ann Oncol* **24**, 2278-2284, doi:10.1093/annonc/mdt182 (2013).

Stearns, V. *et al.* Sentinel lymphadenectomy after neoadjuvant chemotherapy for breast cancer may reliably represent the axilla except for inflammatory breast cancer. *Ann Surg Oncol* **9**, 235-242 (2002).

Sudhan, D. R. *et al.* Extended Adjuvant Therapy with Neratinib Plus Fulvestrant Blocks ER/HER2 Crosstalk and Maintains Complete Responses of ER(+)/HER2(+) Breast Cancers: Implications to the ExteNET Trial. *Clin Cancer Res* **25**, 771-783, doi:10.1158/1078-0432.CCR-18-1131 (2019).

Valeta-Magara, A. *et al.* Inflammatory Breast Cancer Promotes Development of M2 Tumor-associated Macrophages and Cancer Mesenchymal Cells Through a Complex Cytokine Network. *Cancer Res*, doi:10.1158/0008-5472.CAN-17-2158 (2019).

von Minckwitz, G. *et al.* Trastuzumab Emtansine for Residual Invasive HER2-Positive Breast Cancer. *N Engl J Med* **380**, 617-628, doi:10.1056/NEJMoa1814017 (2019).

Walker, G. V. *et al.* Pretreatment staging positron emission tomography/computed tomography in patients with inflammatory breast cancer influences radiation treatment field designs. *International journal of radiation oncology, biology, physics* **83**, 1381-1386, doi:10.1016/j.ijrobp.2011.10.040 (2012).

Wang, D., Feng, J. & Xu, B. A meta-analysis of platinum-based neoadjuvant chemotherapy versus standard neoadjuvant chemotherapy for triple-negative breast cancer. *Future Oncol* **15**, 2779-2790, doi:10.2217/fon-2019-0165 (2019).

Warren, L. E. *et al.* Inflammatory Breast Cancer: Patterns of Failure and the Case for Aggressive Locoregional Management. *Ann Surg Oncol* **22**, 2483-2491, doi:10.1245/s10434-015-4469-4 (2015a).

Warren, L. E. *et al.* Inflammatory breast cancer and development of brain metastases: risk factors and outcomes. *Breast Cancer Res Treat* **151**, 225-232, doi:10.1007/s10549-015-3381-8 (2015b).

Wolfe, A. R. *et al.* Mesenchymal stem cells and macrophages interact through IL-6 to promote inflammatory breast cancer in pre-clinical models. *Oncotarget* **7**, 82482-82492, doi:10.18632/oncotarget.12694 (2016).

Woodward, W. A. *et al.* Scientific Summary from the Morgan Welch MD Anderson Cancer Center Inflammatory Breast Cancer (IBC) Program 10(th) Anniversary Conference. *Journal of Cancer* **8**, 3607-3614, doi:10.7150/jca.21200 (2017).

Woodward, W. A. Postmastectomy radiation therapy for inflammatory breast cancer: is more better? *Int J Radiat Oncol Biol Phys* **89**, 1004-1005, doi:10.1016/j.ijrobp.2014.05.004 (2014).

Zujewski, J. A. & Rubinstein, L. CREATE-X a role for capecitabine in early-stage breast cancer: an analysis of available data. *NPJ Breast Cancer* **3**, 27, doi:10.1038/s41523-017-0029-3 (2017).

4 IBC-Specialized Centers

Naoto T. Ueno, MD, PhD, FACP

Successful elimination of inflammatory breast cancer (IBC) requires implementing a multidisciplinary approach to care of patients with newly diagnosed IBC. It is also important to provide innovative clinical trials to patients with advanced IBC. Over the past five years, we have noticed increasing interest in establishing IBC-specific clinics in the United States (US). For example, Dana-Farber Cancer Institute, Duke University, Cancer Treatment Centers of America in Atlanta, Georgia, and Northwestern University have all recently established IBC clinics. Furthermore, other institutions have announced plans to open centers dedicated to caring for patients with IBC. Having appropriate access points for patients with IBC ensures a high-quality standard of care.

The MD Anderson IBC program, the Morgan Welch Inflammatory Breast Cancer Research Program and Clinic, was established in 2007. It was designed to engage physicians and clinical, translational, and basic-science researchers along with epidemiologists, pathologists, research nurses, clinical coordinators, grant administrators, and support staff within a single administrative infrastructure. The aim of the research program and clinic was to develop a world-class, clinically oriented, translational research–focused IBC program. Our IBC program with multidisciplinary members was envisioned as a network that would design and conduct IBC clinical trials, secure and maintain biospecimens and clinical data resources, and lead the way in creating innovative IBC diagnostic, research, and treatment strategies. Support from the State of Texas afforded the program the capability to build a comprehensive infrastructure to support a dedicated clinical and translational research team, develop specialized IBC resources, and create a portfolio of funded research projects in the laboratory and clinic that would directly improve the overall survival of patients with IBC.

The National Cancer Database shows that trimodality approaches are still not used in 30% to 40% of patients. This is an unfortunate situation because when patients miss surgery, radiation therapy, or systemic therapy, we observe a reduction of the overall survival rate. These data suggest a need to create more IBC-specific clinics and a need for professional education to ensure that healthcare providers understand the standard of care for primary IBC. The past several years of research effort have taught us that the microenvironment has a major impact on IBC. Many researchers have attempted to find a genetic driver that is unique to IBC compared to non-IBC. However, we have yet to find an IBC-specific genetic driver. One may not exist. We have identified genomic characteristics that are associated with IBC, but we have not reached a conclusion that has led to an IBC-specific treatment. Currently, we are actively conducting preclinical and clinical research to improve the rate of pathological complete response to preoperative chemotherapy, with EGFR and JAK2 the two major targets. Further, many investigators are exploring new territory by trying to understand the impact of the cancer microenvironment on IBC. Some research has suggested that macrophage dysregulation and activation of regulatory T cells contribute to the disease process. Many of the new data will help us develop novel targeted therapy or immunotherapy for IBC.

Finally, we have increased the number of IBC-specific clinical trials in the US. Trials offer us research opportunities and offer our patients hope. However, the total number of IBC-specific clinical trials remains in the single digits in the US. Further, there is a need for all IBC clinics to collaborate to design and run IBC-specific clinical trials so that the large numbers of patients will provide robust results. Ultimately, conducting clinical trials is the only way to make advances in the field of IBC.

In the next five years, we will need to better understand the biology of IBC to support preclinical and clinical development of IBC-specific treatment. In particular, we will need to identify the microenvironment changes that drive IBC and the cancer-specific genetic, proteomic, and/or metabolomic changes unique to IBC so that these can be developed as IBC-specific treatment targets or diagnostic tools. Moreover, we will need to ensure that all patients with IBC have access to the best available precision/personalized medical care and treatment. Finally, we will need to determine the molecular risk factors that lead to the development of IBC. This is a lot to accomplish, but this is necessary to enable the progress that we would like to see. We are seeing IBC science and clinical activity increase with the engagement of investigators and the community. Thank you for your wholehearted engagement.

We look forward to being even more productive for patients with IBC in the coming five years!

Part 2:
Patient Stories

Nancy Key

Symptoms

My story starts on a lovely summer day in 1998. I was working in the garden at my daughter's new house when I was bitten on my right side by a common garden spider. I didn't think much about it until the next morning in the shower I noticed a "bug bite" on my right breast, "oh, it got inside my bra" I thought. Days later I noticed the bites on my side were gone but the one on my breast was not. Still, no real concern, even though it itched like crazy. A week or so later, again in the shower, I was aware that the skin around the bump was thick and dimpled like an orange peel. Now that got my attention. I was concerned that it may have been a poison spider and the skin was dying.

Diagnosis

I called my ob/gyn to have it checked and I was scheduled to see her the following week. After a physical exam, she immediately sent me to get a mammogram and ultrasound, even though I had just had a "normal" mammo a couple of months earlier. During the ultrasound, the imaging doctor said that there was a blockage in the lymph system, but he could not determine the cause. More tests would be needed. As I left his office to walk across the hall to my ob/gyn, his nurse took my hand and in a low, serious voice said, "Good luck to you, honey." The hairs on the back of my neck stood on end. My doctor's nurse told me that she had made me an appointment with a surgeon. The next afternoon I met with a lovely young surgeon who took a biopsy of the lymphatic blockage and the thickened skin. She said she would call me with the results. The very next morning her office called and said the doctor wanted to see me that day—July 24—and they advised me to bring my husband. Okay, now I was genuinely worried.

We sat down in her office. She picked up my chart, cleared her throat and said, "I am sorry to tell you that you have breast cancer, and it is unfortunately, the very worst kind." I was reeling. What was she saying? I felt fine, I did self-breast exams regularly, and the was no lump! She explained that this type was called inflammatory breast cancer, or IBC, and the symptoms were radically different from the other types of breast cancer and less common. She told me she had contacted an oncologist whom she respected, and the consultation was the next day, Saturday, on her day off. She described the severity, aggressive behavior, and speed that IBC presented, stressing the need to work diligently and quickly to fight it.

Treatment

The plan was for me to go to the hospital on Monday to begin three days of testing, blood work, EKG, bone scan, cat scan and more. Thursday I was to rest and Friday morning I was back to the hospital to have a port-a-cath surgically inserted for chemotherapy infusions that would begin as soon as I awoke from the anesthesia. I kept thinking "What, there must be some mistake!" She continued to tell me the time frame for my treatment. The first chemo, just one week from that day, would begin a regiment of six rounds of chemo, one every three weeks, followed by a modified radical mastectomy, provided the oncologist was pleased with the effectiveness of the chemo. After a month recovery from that surgery, I'd have six more rounds of a different type of chemo again at three week intervals to be followed by 26 to 30 radiation treatments.

Then she said, "Do you have any questions?" Questions? I didn't even know what half of what she was saying meant, I had never heard of this disease, my head was spinning, and I was sure I was going to faint! My husband scooped me up and we drove home in a deafening silence. He gave me comfort.

The next day, we met my oncologist. She was serious and matter of fact about the next eleven months of my life, letting me know that this was not going to be an easy process and would be fraught with side effects, discomfort, and pain. She advised me not to read about IBC on the Internet or in hard copy, explaining that all I would find was the consensus that I was probably going to die. She did not believe that was the most likely outcome due to the recent changes in protocol and treatment options. She gave me hope.

After the days of testing, my husband and I arrived at the hospital to prep for the outpatient surgery for my port. I was sitting on the side of the bed waiting for the nurse to tell me what to do and I thought about my last few weeks, from a happy housewife working in the garden to a cancer patient shivering and scared. My life and the lives of my family had flipped dramatically. When the nurse came in to begin my IV, I was washed over by a wave of terror. This was real. It wasn't a mistake! I silently wept. The nurse took my hand and squeezed. She gave me strength.

Response to Treatment

So the routine began, chemo infusions that took between four and five hours, then home to rest. About five hours after the completion of the chemo I was overwhelmed with nausea. It would come in waves about once an hour. If I moved around at all, it hit again, so I spent the majority of my time on the couch or in the bathroom. The oral nausea medication they gave me was promptly thrown up. The only help was suppositories, which were of minimal relief. The second week was better, I didn't throw up as much, but it did feel like I was in a boat in the middle of the perfect storm. This week at least I could eat a little, but something in the chemo made my mouth sore and everything I tried to eat tasted metallic. But most of what I could force down stayed down. The third week was pretty good, not much nausea, and a tiny flicker of energy, but I knew that more chemo was only a few days away! I was overwhelmed and sure I had ruined my family's lives. I could no longer care for my three year old grandson, my daughter had to hurriedly find adequate daycare, my husband was stressed and scared, and it was all my fault. I wasn't sure I was going to be able to do it. Seventeen days into my first round of chemo in the middle of the night, the house was cold and dark and silent. My husband was sleeping. I had taken a pillow and blanket into the bathroom so I didn't disturb him, since I was in there most of the time anyway.

A Change in Attitude

As I laid my head on the side of the tub to try to rest after puking and crying, it dawned on me. I had to take control of this! I began to think of ways I could do that. I couldn't do anything about the drugs and side effects, so why not think of them in a different way. I decided to see vomiting as throwing up cancer cells, my hair was falling out so that meant the chemo was working, my energy was gone because my body was busy killing cancer. Surprisingly that decision changed a lot for me emotionally. I gave myself perseverance.

Complications

One morning, after my second round of chemo, I awoke to a severely swollen arm. It was so swollen that the skin was tight. It looked like a giant sausage. I drove myself to the cancer center, which was only three minutes from my house, I had a blood work appointment anyway. When I walked in you would have thought I had an axe in my head. Everyone began to run around me, talking rapidly, putting me in a wheel chair and rushing me to ICU. I had developed a blood clot on the end of the tube of the port a cath. I spend a day getting special treatments to reduce the clot, spent the night in the hospital with my arm wrapped in ice, and the next morning had the old port taken out and a new one put in a larger artery. After this short break the mundane process resumed.

The chemo routine went on for about three months. Each time before my next round the oncologist would ask if I wanted her to reduce the dosage. I was pretty sure I could survive the treatments, and I was very sure I could not survive the disease, so I never backed it down.

Surgery

I met with the surgeon to consult about the mastectomy, I wanted her to cut off both of my breasts. That seemed logical and easier than dealing with a prosthesis every time I would be with people. She disagreed, stating that she was going to take lymph nodes from the cancer side, and really didn't want to disturb the ones on the other side. I fought for my plan but she convinced me it was wiser to get a breast reduction instead. So I met with a plastic surgeon for that procedure. I explained to him that I wanted to be as small as I could, flat even, he insisted that he would make my breast pretty and symmetrical, in case I wanted reconstruction on the other side in the future. I did not. My docs had told me not to ever cover the site because recurrence is likely with IBC. The surgeries were performed at the same time and when I awakened from them my surgeon was standing next to my bed holding my hand. She said, "Doesn't it feel good to know the cancer is gone." I spent the next four weeks with drains and exercises but I felt pretty good without the chemo.

A New Treatment

The next three months were a different type of chemo drug. This one didn't upset my stomach, but it made my bones ache. For three days before each infusion I had to take a steroid, so my body would accept the chemo. That steroid made me feel schizophrenic, like I was about to jump out of my skin, but too tired to move. My eyes jiggled, so reading was out, TV was marginal. I just closed my eyes and listened. But mostly this chemo made me tired and achy. It would hurt to watch my husband walk. Again I spent my time on the couch.

When chemo was finished I began radiation. I did not know what to expect, but the kindest doctor guided me through the process with grace. These treatments were every week day for six weeks. They sapped my energy and blistered my skin, but with a calm stomach they were tolerable. On the day of my last radiation the staff brought a placard and balloons to commemorate my completion of treatment. I was thrilled, and yet frightened. What would I do now? Who would I talk with for my questions? I could not just go back to my previous life, I was not the same person. I asked my doc and she said, "Go live your life." I had no idea what that meant. She gave me possibilities.

A New Lease on Life

About half way through my treatment I joined a support group for breast cancer. The ladies were understanding and helpful, and we often ended up in bouts of laughter. These survivors taught me that there was life after all this mayhem, and it could be a darn good one, just not the one I had before. By the time my treatment was over I was sure that these lovely sisters of breast cancer were the most alive people that I had ever known, and I wanted to be that too. I can honestly say that my life now is better, different yes, but better than it has ever been. I appreciate each day, have truly learned how to play and love more preciously than when I was "normal." I am aware every day how lucky I am that I survived this horrid disease. I have attended too many funerals of lovely women that I have met on this journey to ever forget. I am vigilant of my health, staying fit and helping my immune system function as efficiently as possible. I am sure that I have survived due to the fact that my doctor knew what IBC was from the very beginning and rushed me into treatment. She gave me life.

I wrote the words above six years ago, and I am only days away from celebrating my twenty-second cancerversary. We always do something special—my husband never forgets— taking me out to dinner or presenting me with a single flower.

I have been accused of being a "Polly Anna" with my happy, upbeat attitude. I am honored at that moniker, I am blessed to be alive, and I continue to remember my gratitude. After facing "the devil cancer," I simply do not have the time to put any of my energy on negative things or people. I am smarter than I knew before all this, much stronger than I ever realized, and happier than I could have imagined after this diagnosis. My life is rich with joy, laughter, and discover. Cancer gave me a new perspective.

Christine Paroz

Diagnosis

My life changed irrevocably in ways you don't wish upon anyone when I was diagnosed with IBC in May of 2005. I knew within myself that I had a problem with my right breast as it was so swollen and red. I decided to see a breast surgeon in Brisbane, about a two hour drive from Toowoomba, Australia, where I live. This beautiful surgeon, whose name is Teresa, took so much time with me, and she said, "You have inflammatory breast cancer," and she had only seen a limited number of cases before, so my journey began.

Treatment

I started chemo soon after, which I had for three months. It was supposed to shrink the tumour, which was 85 mm, but it did not. Then came my surgery, a full mastectomy plus the lymph nodes, which were all cancerous. Following surgery I was told that I had to have more chemo (Adriamycin, Cyclophosphamide, and Docetaxel) and radium, and that I was HER2 positive.[164] So my oncologist asked the board at the hospital if I would be eligible

---

164 HER2 positive means that the patient has the HER2 receptor on the tumor, which can be targeted to diminish replication of tumor cells. Herceptin does not kill cancer cells. Rather, it inhibits their growth.

for the trial drug Herceptin. I was lucky enough to be granted the drug and I still have it today.

Aftermath

I suffer badly from lymphoedema (obstruction of the lymphatic channel, causing the arm to swell) and over the years have spent a few times in hospital with infections as well as swelling, for which a compression bandage is applied. So this is my story about my journey with IBC. I thank my wonderful surgeon Teresa and my oncologist for their ongoing care. I will be forever grateful to them.

Current Treatment

I have stayed on Herceptin for 15 years and will continue to do so indefinitely. It certainly has been a wonder drug for me. So I am still doing well. I have issues with lymphedema, for which I wear a compression sleeve, but I am so thankful I am here and I proudly say I am a survivor of IBC.

Kathy Patton

My Breast Cancer Stories

My first breast cancer story began in early December of 1999, when I was 46 years old. The real fun doesn't begin until 2005 so please read on. Now, back to my December 1999 episode. I had an ultrasound done so the radiologist would know where to insert the needle in order for the breast surgeon to take a biopsy. Once the radiologist placed the needle in my left breast, he followed up by placing a small foam cup on top of the needle and taping it to my skin to make sure the needle would not move. I was wheeled into the Operating Room, put to sleep and before I knew it, the procedure was over. I received a call for an appointment to see the breast surgeon for the results of my biopsy. He told me it was benign and I was soooo relieved, however, he then mentioned to me that I needed to have a mammogram in six weeks, just to be on the safe side. In all honesty, I looked at him as if he had two heads. I told him I thought that was very strange, but he just shrugged it off and told me, he tells all his patients the same thing; better safe than sorry. I was not impressed! When I heard those words come out of his mouth, I wasn't feeling very secure at that point. However, I followed his advice and had a mammogram, and the radiologist on site that day called me in and magnified my films along with circling the areas that looked suspicious. The radiologist told me these suspicious-looking micro-calcification deposits had never been removed.

First Cancer Diagnosis

Now, I'll begin my next chapter. This radiologist was very knowledgeable and experienced; maybe he had seen and dealt with so many various types of breast cancer in his years of practicing. He was very close to retirement but still so incredibly dedicated. I felt very safe with this man. He told me he wanted to perform a stereotactic biopsy on me and he felt sure he could get a piece of the micro-calcification deposit to be biopsied. I agreed and went to a new facility along with getting a new breast surgeon and breast oncologist. When the radiologist performed the stereotactic biopsy, I had to lay flat on a stretcher, face down, and my left breast hung through a hole in the stretcher. Even though the radiologist was trying to numb me, he had to go so deep that it was extremely painful, but I am very grateful to him because he was successful in getting a piece to biopsy.

The radiologist told me specifically that he would call me on Wednesday, February 1, 2000, at 3 pm to let me know what I was dealing with at this time. Well, at exactly 3 pm on Wednesday, the phone rang and it was the radiologist informing me that it was breast cancer; however, the good news was this was the earliest possible stage of breast cancer. I was diagnosed with non-invasive ductal carcinoma in situ, stage 0, which is micro-calcification deposits in the duct of my left breast. I was told at least 80 to 85 percent of people with micro-calcification deposits are pre-cancer, but that was not the case with me. I met my new breast oncologist and new breast surgeon, who I liked very much. My new breast surgeon performed a surgical lumpectomy. This time there was no needle fiasco like the first incident back in December 1999. The results came back, and even though the breast surgeon got it all, my breast oncologist wanted him to widen the margins to be on the safe side, which my breast surgeon did the following month. Since my cancer was non-invasive, I didn't need chemotherapy, only radiation. I had

33 treatments of radiation on my left breast, and my only side effect, as a result of the radiation, was the dryness of my skin around the fourth week.

Once the radiation was complete, the next step was tamoxifen. My breast oncologist wanted me to stay on tamoxifen for five years. At that time, I was working as an executive assistant for the CFO and CIO of the fourth largest healthcare organization in the country, so I had to always be sharp as a tack, which was never a problem in the past. The tamoxifen wasn't allowing me to be on top of my game, and by the sixth week, I had extreme difficulty concentrating, and as a result, my breast oncologist took me off tamoxifen. I stressed to her my concern about replacing the tamoxifen with another drug so I wouldn't have any kind of recurrence. The oncologist told me, "You are cured; you have no worries."
Now the nightmare begins...

New Symptoms

I went two months shy of six years being considered cancer-free. That changed on a night I will never forget. It was a work night and all that was above my left breast, prior to retiring for the evening, was a straight three-inch scar line from the several lumpectomies I had done when diagnosed with my first breast cancer in 2000. I woke up the next morning and my left breast, the same breast that had the first breast cancer, was twice normal size, red, very hard to the touch, warm, with an inverted nipple that was slightly black and blue along the outside of my left breast and with a peau d'orange effect below the nipple. The skin below the nipple also looked rather thick. I couldn't imagine what this could be.

Initial Treatment

My husband, Russ, and I went to my primary care physician and she placed me on an antibiotic for mastitis. I had a gut feeling that she knew what was going on but wouldn't tell me. The only thing she did tell me was that if my left breast didn't greatly improve within three to five days, I needed to see my breast oncologist and breast surgeon. Unfortunately, my breast didn't improve at all, so my husband and I headed to my breast oncologist, the doctor who had told me, "You are cured; you have no worries."

Second Cancer Diagnosis

When she took a look at my left breast, her face turned as white as a sheet. She immediately left the room, and when she returned, she told me to please go down to pre-admission testing quickly, as it was 4 pm when this took place. She concluded her conversation by telling me that I was scheduled for a biopsy at 8 am the following morning, on December 1, 2005.

I asked her what was I dealing with but she wasn't sure. Again, my gut told me she knew. My husband went with me to get the results of the biopsy on December 8, 2005.

The breast surgeon was in the same building as my breast oncologist, which made it much more convenient. When I received the news that the biopsy confirmed I had inflammatory breast cancer (IBC), stage III, in the same breast as my first breast cancer, I dropped to my knees. I was in total shock!!!

My husband and I ran directly to my breast oncologist's office, and without an appointment, she took me immediately. She ordered various tests to see if the cancer metastasized, which it didn't, thank goodness! My breast oncologist shipped all my test reports to the Center City Philadelphia Hospital and gave me my films to take there the following Monday. My breast oncologist also set up everything for me. All I had to do was show up.

When I met my new Center City Philadelphia breast oncologist, my very first question to her was, "Is this a death sentence?" She responded immediately that she felt it wasn't. When I think of it now, I really don't know what she thought, but I really did appreciate her response at that time.

I was placed in a clinical trial at that time starting the week of December 12; four MRIs would be scheduled during this trial.

Treatment

The week of December 12, 2005 I was infused with the first chemotherapy regime of Adriamycin and Cytoxan (A/C). Since the doctors moved so quickly with me, my port-a-cath wasn't placed in my chest until the following Monday. I was given this chemotherapy at four different intervals on a bi-weekly basis for two months. Unfortunately, by the time I was to receive my third A/C treatment, I was so sick and feverish that my husband took me back to my Center City Philadelphia oncologist. When my breast oncologist saw me, my white cell count was marginal. I had developed neutropenic fever and while in the hospital for six days, I contracted the C-Diff bacterial infection, which I've had at least four times since that occurrence.

Once I had completed the four A/C cycles of treatment, I started getting infused with Taxol on a weekly basis, which was suppose to last 12 weeks but in my case, it only lasted 11 weeks because the MRI showed that my IBC was contained, and once the doctors can contain the IBC, a person is ready for surgery.

Since my modified radical mastectomy (left breast) and simple mastectomy (right breast) were originally scheduled for June 15, 2006, I wanted the surgery pushed up immediately. As a result of my hysteria, the surgery was performed on May 11, 2006. I was in the Center City Philadelphia Hospital for two nights and went home with three drains, which lasted ten days until my Center City Philadelphia breast surgeon removed them. I never had breast reconstruction.

As my journey continues with IBC, various complications have arisen, which have caused five bouts of cellulitis. In July 2006, my breast oncologist told me I had no evidence of disease (NED), however, my husband and I felt somewhat uncomfortable with this diagnosis. We felt more should be done. My breast oncologist placed me on a chemotherapy drug called vinorelbine (Navelbine). I think she did this just so I would feel more comfortable.

While I was receiving several months of chemotherapy prior to my mastectomies, my husband was researching the Internet to find a breast oncologist that had the most experience with this aggressive, lethal form of breast cancer, because IBC is not usually detected by mammograms and ultrasounds, and you don't have to have a lump. I was completely unaware that my husband was doing any type of research, but I am so incredibly thankful.

New Physician

My husband found a breast oncologist that was extremely knowledgeable in the area of IBC. His name is Dr. Massimo Cristofanilli, or Dr. C, which I like to call him. At that time Dr. C was located at MD Anderson Cancer Center in Houston, Texas. On August 8, 2006, my husband and I met Dr. C. We were both impressed and knew we had made the right decision. Dr. Cristofanilli immediately took me off Navelbine, as he didn't feel it was necessary at this time. During my first visit with Dr. Cristofanilli, he did four days of extensive testing; more testing than the Center City Philadelphia Hospital ever did. The Center City Philadelphia Hospital refused to do a PET Scan on me because I was told by my breast oncologist that it wasn't their protocol for IBC.

My husband and I continued to fly to MD Anderson in Houston, Texas every three months from August 2006 until December 2009, and I had a PET scan done at each visit. Dr. C informed me that he was relocating to Fox Chase Cancer Center in Northeast Philadelphia as of January 2010. I was amazed and knew right then and there that Father God truly does work in mysterious ways.

First Recurrence and Treatment

Since my initial diagnosis of IBC, I've experienced two recurrences. My first recurrence took place in September 2007. I noticed a small piece of skin that almost looked like a skin tag. Since I was back in the Philadelphia area, I went to my breast oncologist and she sent me to my breast surgeon. I had a gut feeling that something was really wrong and I wanted this gone! My breast surgeon took out the very tiny piece of skin, and on Sept. 27, 2007 called to tell me it was cancer from the IBC.

My breast oncologist asked the surgeon to make the margins wider, which he did. Once this was completed, my breast oncologist notified Dr. C at MD Anderson in Houston, Texas, as I had requested that she keep him posted regularly. I asked her if she would please follow Dr. Cristofanilli's instructions, and she agreed to do so. She did say that if she disagreed with his instructions, she would let me know; however, she would still follow his instructions. I was very grateful for her understanding.

The Center City Philadelphia Hospital told me that once again I was NED. I already had an appointment scheduled with Dr. Cristofanilli, but once my Center City Philadelphia breast oncologist told Dr. Cristofanilli about my surgery, he wanted to see me as soon as possible.

In December 2007, my husband and I met with Dr. Cristofanilli. He was extremely concerned and not pleased that I had this surgery performed. He asked me why I had done this, and I told him I was extremely worried and all the doctors told me it was nothing. Dr. Cristofanilli stressed to me when you have IBC, you never want to upset the applecart. I told him I would follow his directions from that point on. I admit my fear did get the best of me.

Second Recurrence and Treatment

I was so thankful that I was at MD Anderson in Houston, Texas, because they did more extensive testing than the Center City Philadelphia Hospital did, and I found out that I was, in fact, not NED, as I had two abnormal lymph nodes in my right axilla area (armpit), which indicated another recurrence of IBC. As a result of this finding, I was considered stage IV. Sometimes I wonder if it was another recurrence or was always there, but since the Center City Philadelphia Hospital never checked, how would I know?

I fought this recurrence with chemotherapy and Herceptin from December 2007 until December 2010, when Dr. Cristofanilli told me he was stopping the chemotherapy and wanted me to have radiation, which I did.

Response to Second Treatment

The entire time I was battling these two nodes in my right axilla area with chemotherapy and Herceptin at Fox Chase Cancer Center, they would sometimes get smaller and sometimes larger, as all the PET scans showed, but they never completely went away. I was very impressed with the radiation department at Fox Chase Cancer Center. They were extremely thorough. I ended up having 25 treatments of my right supraclavicular area, which is aligned with my right axilla area.

Since we were fighting the two nodes in my right axilla area, the next 8 treatments were boost treatments strictly directed at the nodes in my right axilla area. The 33 radiation treatments on my right side were completed on January 28, 2011. The following PET scan showed that the nodes were gone and it looked like all was clear after battling this recurrence for three years and two months.

Ups and Downs Through the Years

Since 2011, there have been times my PET scans were clear! However, I've also dealt with several flare-ups of IBC as well as cellulitis bouts, where I needed to be hospitalized to receive an IV antibiotic. Dr. C had placed me in at least four studies, which help all patients as well as those in the studies. I've been on various chemotherapies and drugs. I've also had the Guardant360 liquid biopsy, which provides a comprehensive molecular analysis of the cancer cells.

My PET scan at Northwestern Memorial Hospital in August 2016 showed a small cancerous lymph node. Since my left breast area has had stubborn nodes at various times, Dr. C contacted the radiation oncologist at the Center City Philadelphia Hospital to arrange for brachytherapy, which delivers radiation directly to a small area around the surgery site and does not treat the entire breast. The goal is to limit side effects of radiation to normal tissue. I started brachytherapy on August 16, 2016 and was treated once per week for six weeks.

In December 2017, my PET scan showed a skin recurrence of IBC in the same area where punch biopsies and the previous brachytherapy was done. Dr. C and the radiation oncologist decided that I could have brachytherapy again plus hyperthermia treatments, which is performed with heat. The brachytherapy treatments ended in February 2018. I stopped the hyperthermia treatments earlier as they were too painful. As time went on, I started to develop a hole where the brachytherapy was performed. I needed help with this so a nurse from Mercy Home Health came by my home frequently to pack the hole. Finally I started packing the hole myself, but it got deeper and deeper. I packed it for seven months because the vascular surgeon told me to live with it, which was unbelievable! However, I had surgery for the hole by a breast/plastic surgeon at the Center City Philadelphia Hospital on September 18, 2018. By then the hole was deep enough to see a little bone. Since the hole was the result of radiation damage, the surgeon created a flap that was much larger than the hole to ensure the skin would stay together. The surgeon informed me after the surgery that one of my ribs was black and broken. This surgeon did an excellent job. I was so grateful and relieved. After that, I never wrote in my journal again.

As a result of my PET scan at Northwestern on Feb. 24, 2020, Dr. C decided to keep me on Aromasin (exemstane) hormone treatment. I've been on this drug in the past, but the cancer has returned. Whenever I had a PET scan in Chicago, Dr. C would meet with my husband and me to go over the images so I knew exactly what I was dealing with. I'm so thankful for Dr. C.

I had a PET at Jefferson Hospital in Philadelphia on August 1, 2020. It wasn't clear, but I don't know exactly what's going on yet. Due to the pandemic, I will be sending the CD of this PET scan plus the report to Dr. C at Northwestern in Chicago so he can discuss the results with my local oncologist.

I will be on some type of medication or treatment of some kind for the rest of my life, and I'm very ok with this, because I realize how blessed I have been.

Lessons Learned

The most important lesson I've learned from all of this is: if you are fortunate enough to have good healthcare insurance, as well as access to a top-notch facility with top-notch physicians that have extensive experience with the type of cancer you are battling—especially when it is rare, aggressive, and lethal—you must do it because it truly is a matter of life or death.

Since my very first breast cancer began back in 1999, I've kept a journal. I have 14 journals and would have more, but I stopped after the surgery to repair the hole in the left side of my chest. Journaling helped me keep track of my somewhat crazy life over the last several years. Journaling is a very good tool to use especially when you deal with chemobrain.

When I think back since my initial diagnosis with IBC in 2005, I thank Father God every day for Dr. Massimo Cristofanilli. I truly believe my Dr. C is my angel here on earth.

Pat Shodean

My IBC Journey

The first week of December, 1997, I was vacationing in Florida with my new husband. We had married the previous August of 1996. This was to be our delayed honeymoon. We went for a friend's wedding and made plans for touring the sites around Orlando. I was 51 years old and post-menopausal, having had a hysterectomy in 1989. I had also been doing hormone replacement therapy since the hysterectomy. This, according to my surgeon, "fed" my cancer for the past eight years.

Symptoms

While in Florida, I noticed my breast suddenly became swollen, red, and "hot." By the next day I could feel a soft lump in the upper, outer quadrant of my right breast. I thought it was an infection or blocked duct and didn't want anything to spoil our fun times in Florida.

Initial Treatment

I went to a local walk-in clinic for an antibiotic. That is exactly what they prescribed, and they also believed it was indeed an infection or mastitis. I was also instructed to use hot compresses on the area. The swelling and soreness improved, but only slightly. We continued to enjoy our vacation, but I was worried even though I had heard that cancer doesn't hurt!

Second Treatment

We returned to Albuquerque the following week, and I finished taking the prescribed antibiotic. The swelling and soreness were better, but not gone. I went to my primary care physician who recommended I see a breast specialist right away. He told me later that he suspected IBC, but had only read about it and had not actually seen it in a patient. At that time I worked for a group of radiology physicians and knew of a specialist they worked with. I was able to get an appointment right away because she knew me. She prescribed a second antibiotic, but it didn't work either.

Additional Symptoms

By Christmas week the lymph glands under my arm were also swollen and sore. The specialist/surgeon did a core biopsy the day after Christmas—not quite four weeks after initial symptoms. She also ordered a mammogram and an ultrasound. Since I worked for the radiology group, I did not have to wait for appointments for these tests or for their results. (I had previously had a mammogram in June of that year, which was normal.) The results of both of these new tests were unremarkable.

Diagnosis

When I went back for the results of the biopsy, the breast specialist told me, "It's cancer and a bad one!" My breast doctor is not much on bedside manner, or the touchy-feely stuff, but I knew she was a strong advocate for her patients—one of the reasons I chose her, and she was considered an expert in her field.

The following Monday I had a breast MRI, bone scan, and other tests I can't even remember. Back then a breast MRI was fairly new and our radiology group was just starting to do them. One of the radiologists showed me the results that day and explained that some women with IBC don't get diagnosed for six months. The MRI did show the cancer growing in sheets on the surface of the breast. Several times during my testing day members of my radiology group called to check on me and consult with the testing physicians and technicians.

A New Treatment

Needless to say I was devastated! My husband's first wife had died from breast cancer metastases and we were both in shock. Only a week later, New Year's Eve, we were in the office of the oncologist laying out a treatment plan. He also had received several phone calls relative to my diagnosis and treatment. My oncologist felt the treatment should be very aggressive since my cancer was aggressive. He also recommended that we include a stem cell transplant as part of my treatment plan. I had never heard of this and received a full explanation, part of that being a required pre-authorization from my health plan. Happy New Year!

I have three grown children and one of the really hardest parts of this whole ordeal was making the phone calls the next day to say, "Hi, kids. I hope your New Year is terrific and by the way I'm starting chemo for cancer tomorrow!"

The first week of January 1998, a double Hickman catheter was surgically implanted in my upper chest area and I started my first round of Cytoxan, Adriamycin and Fluorouracil chemotherapy (CAF chemo). We learned to love that catheter, and I lived with it for seven months. We became experts at flushing it every morning and every night. Initially, I could just tuck the two ends into my bra so they didn't flop around, but after the mastectomy, that wasn't workable since I no longer wore a bra. I developed the method of taping tabs on the catheter tips, and using a big safety pin, I attached the tips with the pin to a soft cotton jersey loop I made for around my neck. Since I have always had difficult veins (they roll and collapse), I was grateful not to be repeatedly stuck over the next months of treatment.

Today I sometimes wish I could have that catheter back since it made administering the chemo meds and drawing blood so simple and painless. I had four rounds of chemo, two weeks apart (called dose-dense). My blood counts stayed pretty consistent with the predictions for crashing and recovering. Luckily I never had to delay a chemo session due to low blood counts. In fact, I didn't have to sit all day for infusions. My chemo was administered using a 24-hour pump in a fanny pack that I wore at home and returned the next day when the treatment was completed. I just threw that bugger up on the headboard at night and hoped I didn't get tangled in the tubing.

I was mobile for those infusion days and could go to lunch and visit my mother and sister, who were very supportive. One way I was able to count down the time was to think in percentages—25 percent done, 50 percent done, etc. I'm guessing that it was my shopping/sale calculation mentality that helped me through this period and plan for the next steps.

Response to Treatment

In anticipation of my hair falling out, I asked my sister to give me a buzz cut. I thought that the bald Sigourney Weaver looked pretty good in the *Alien* movie and that's what I thought I would see in the mirror. Unfortunately, I looked more like Rod Steiger! We both had a good cry at this emotional time. I'm not sure cutting my hair short was the wisest thing to do because sleeping became painful on my scalp—kind of like when you wore a ponytail too tight and your hair follicles got sore. Anyway my hair fell out after the second chemo treatment. I wore wigs and scarves when I went out but was most comfortable just being a baldy at home. I live in a desert climate, where spring and summer get hot. I do recall that my head would get cold at night so I sometimes wore a soft knit cap to bed.

I continued to work part time. I was employed by a group of 18 physicians who were very understanding and flexible about my side effects and energy levels. Sometimes I would consult with them for opinions and some consoling. In fact, one of our doctors, a female, told me that if she were sick and had what I had, she would have chosen the same specialists.

The prescribed medications kept me from being nauseous, but I did have alternating constipation and diarrhea. Some of the side effects I endured were the loss of toenails and fingernails and spidering of the veins in my legs, ankles, and feet. I developed some type of intestinal infection around April 15, which hospitalized me with a fever for a few days. The only good part of that event was that I had just completed our tax returns and it was now up to my husband to get to the post office before 10 p.m. He called to tell me that they served coffee and cookies to the late filers! I told him not to count on that for the next year!

My younger brother was a great help to me during this time, explaining side effects and helpful ways to counter them since he had gone through chemo the year before me for non-Hodgkin's lymphoma. He suggested writing a diary or journal recording treatments and side effects so I could actually plan my life and work around them. We also discussed whether there was some genetic link to our cancers. Our respective oncologists did not believe this was a factor in our diagnoses. We just had bad luck.

My techie brother-in-law had found the Erase IBC website early on, but I wasn't up to reading much of the information and never posted. I just lurked for a long while. Later I discovered that the website was a great information source and an activity I could do in the wee hours of the morning when I couldn't sleep, even though focusing my eyes was a challenge, and mentally keeping a train of thought was difficult too. I recall sometime during my surfing that my treatment protocol was exactly what others were recommending. My thoughts of obtaining a second opinion were resolved, knowing I was on the right track.

I learned that one symptom many IBC'ers related was intense itching of the affected breast before diagnosis. I remembered the previous summer complaining to my mother that something was making my right breast itch like crazy in the nipple area. She suggested changing soap or changing to a different bra. The itching eventually went away. Little did we know that this could have been a preliminary indication of the cancer beginning.

Chemo-brain is not a made up thing. It happens, and gradually my thought processes returned. My daughter bought me a coloring book and oddly that was a wonderfully soothing pastime that I have often recommended to others. The chemo makes you feel like a blob. You don't want to do anything...not sit, lie down, eat, or be sociable. You just are there...waiting to feel better. I even asked the oncologist if I could have a margarita, a favorite cocktail of mine. He said he couldn't believe I actually wanted a margarita. I said, "I just want to feel normal!"

When I got really depressed, it dawned on me one day that I was a lot better off than Christopher Reeve, who had just been thrown from his horse and was paralyzed from the neck down. I didn't have it so bad. You can always find someone who is worse off than you are. Somehow that comparison put things more in perspective and made them easier to accept.

There were days when I wondered whether I really did have cancer...maybe it was all a big mistake and I was being tortured for nothing! (There is no explanation for how your brain waves ricochet around in your head. Well, my brain, anyway.)

Surgery

In early May, I had a modified radical mastectomy of the right breast. The surgery was not difficult. In fact, I had it at 5:00 p.m. one evening and went home the next morning. The surgeon told me since I had no kids at home and had a husband to help me, I should go home to recuperate. She said, "People get sick in hospitals!" I felt so good that we stopped to eat lunch on the way home. I was still numb and wrapped pretty tightly, and I was very hungry! The breast surgeon was fanatical about exercises and regaining full use of my right arm. She threatened me with physical therapy if I couldn't raise my arm straight over my head so my bicep touched my ear. Some days were pretty uncomfortable trying to do this, especially when you could hear and feel the scar tissue tearing loose, but I did it and still have pretty much a full range of motion in my right arm.

Complications

It was at this time we discovered I was allergic to the adhesive tape used to cover the incisions. When the tape was removed, the skin came off with it making the area very sore and scabby. From this point forward, I brought my own paper tape to everything! It's not generally stocked, due to the increased cost. We also discovered the beginnings of lymphedema in my extremely dominant right arm. The surgeon did not think it amounted to anything; however as the years progressed, so did the swelling, pain, and future treatments. I still require compression garments and do manual lymph drainage when my arm gets uncomfortable and swollen. I've adapted my life and wardrobe to accommodate the limitations for this arm. I didn't bowl much or toss horseshoes, but now that I shouldn't, of course, I wanted to do those things.

One thing I discovered that really surprised me was that when I asked our medical director to decipher the lab report after my mastectomy, the first thing he did was look at the top of the report to see who the technician was. He said, "She's a good one!" Naturally, my immediate thought was what would he say if she weren't "a good one." I was pretty sure I understood what was described in the pathology report about the specimens and biopsies, but I wanted a straightforward, honest second opinion of the report's content and ramifications.

Another time of amazing thankfulness I remember was when the hospital radiology department called and left a message on my home phone that there was a question about my latest chest X-ray. I was working and didn't get the message until after work hours on a Friday night. Of course, I was in a panic, assuming that the cancer had spread to my lungs, and I knew I could not last until Monday to find out what the problem was. Thank God one of my radiologists that I knew quite well was working that night. I called him and asked that he look at my X-ray. He invited me down to the hospital, re-took the X-ray, and gave me a big hug and words of encouragement. The previous questionable film just showed a slight shadow that turned out to be nothing. Another "whew" in my journey, but some resentment that whoever left the message did not understand the unnecessary worry they had caused.

In the middle of all this we closed on a new house. We had debated continuing with the purchase, due to my diagnosis, but we focused on the positive and went ahead with it. I was limited in the use of my right arm and was extremely fatigued, but we were blessed to have a wonderful church family that moved us and my sister helpfully set up my kitchen. Unfortunately, she's left-handed, and it took me another year to get everything sorted out. I felt guilty and sad that I had let my husband down by his having to repeat being the caregiver to a breast cancer patient. He told me he was in my life for a reason and he had already seen a bald, one-breasted woman. He was not shocked and was a great medical assistant to me and was a cheerful and encouraging caregiver. I had the drains in for only ten days and wore large shirts without a bra. I was a 38-40 DD so the shirts were very large! I continued to work when I could. My office offered earned sick days for their employees. Many of them donated their sick time to me so I never had to take time off without pay until I had my stem cell transplant.

Sometime during my early treatment, I went to the Social Security office and applied for disability benefits. The person who took my application indicated my type of cancer was an automatic approval, and she also backdated my application to the date of diagnosis, which shortened the usual six-month waiting period.

Stem Cell Transplant and Response

In June I began high dose chemo in preparation for the stem cell transplant. This was the most difficult part of my treatment, although I was hospitalized for only 16 days. It was the only time I experienced mouth sores and a very painful intestinal infection. The little fuzz that had regrown on my head was now gone. No hair again. I also had a painful angina attack while in the hospital, but did not have any cardiac repercussions. It felt like I had a huge boulder on my chest, it was quite painful, and I could hardly breathe. When I alerted the nurse, she was quick to call my doctor, who in turn got a cardiologist to me right away. This must have been a big concern because at other times I found the hospital staff not so quick to respond.

I was told that there would be a stress test the next day. I said, "You actually expect me to get up and walk on a treadmill?" No, thank goodness, they were able to do the test chemically while I was lying down. During my treatments, I had to take Neupogen shots to activate the baby bone marrow cells. After the first two shots, which were administered in the oncologist's office in the mornings before I went to work, I experienced such severe bone pain and general aching that I was unable to function during the day. I was not able to continue working due to the pain.

My blood counts were good enough that the risk of infection was minimal. When I consulted my brother, he recommended that we get permission to give the shots ourselves at home. He found that when he needed Neupogen shots, he gave the shots to himself at night, took a sleeping pill and Tylenol, and then slept through the worst of the side effects. So my husband gave me the injections in the evenings just before dinnertime. By the time the side effects kicked in, I took the Tylenol and a sleeping pill and slept through most of the side effects. Why didn't the oncologist know about this method? It really worked, and so could I—part time. I would certainly recommend this method to anyone who has to take those nasty Neupogen shots. The actual shot part in the stomach was fairly simple and painless. Another hint—make sure the alcohol swipe completely dries before inserting the needle. Then the shot doesn't sting.

I was hospitalized in anticipation of the stem cell transplant and received extremely high doses of chemo. Then there was time for recovery in a clean room with limited visitors because my body had no resistance to infection. Funny, I noticed the same bug in the ceiling light fixture the whole time. It wasn't moving and I took that as a good sign. I had tubes implanted in my neck to prepare for the harvesting and reinfusion of the stem cells. As soon as my blood count was high enough, the baby cells were harvested and frozen. Many of my friends, family, and coworkers donated blood platelets for me. In fact, one young woman came to me tearfully to say she did not weigh enough (evidently 100 pounds was required), so her mother was donating platelets for me on her behalf. Later the blood bank called and asked if they could release the extra platelets to other patients. They had received a very large amount donated in my name. What an affirmation of caring from family, friends, and coworkers! As soon as I had enough white blood cells to fight off infections, I was sent home to recuperate.

When I was released from the hospital, I went directly to my gynecologist and asked that he see me immediately. Who could turn down a sobbing, bald woman with tubes coming out of her neck? I suffered from what I found out was a painful yeast infection during my time in the hospital, enduring awful vaginal sores that made it impossible to walk, sit, or lie on my side. While hospitalized I was given ice packs to relieve the symptoms of these sores. I also had sores in my mouth, and my throat felt like I was being strangled. The gynecologist recognized immediately what this was and was able to treat my condition.

I just wished the oncologist had recommended something weeks before. When he came into my room on his rounds, I would throw back the sheet and point to my groin area and say, "Look at this!" He told me he had never seen a reaction like that to the high dose chemo. He didn't mean my reaction, but the sores. There was no body hair on me due to the chemo, so the sores were very visible. I guess some things were just out of his field of expertise because in every other way, he was and still is wonderful. Gradually over the years my appointments decreased from three-month to six-month intervals, and I have just been put on an annual appointment schedule.

The chemo drugs affected my mind, eyesight, attitude, energy and every part of my being. Fighting the mental anguish is as big an effort as fighting the side effects of the drugs. Everyone was very proud that I have survived such an onslaught to my body. They tell me how good I look whether I do or not. I understand that many people—family and friends included—just don't know what to say. I have an older brother who didn't talk to me for a year. He said he just didn't know what to say although he did talk with my sister and mother, checking up on me. I know a lot of women think, "Wow, I'm glad it's her and not me!" I remember that's what I used to think. It's daunting to realize that now I am living every woman's nightmare.

Further Treatments

I began taking tamoxifen sometime during that summer and tolerated the joint pain pretty well for three years. Then the oncologist switched me to Femara, which was kinder to my body. I stayed on Femara for the next eight years (and battled my insurance company to keep it on their lower tier for co-pays, although I was not successful). The cost of that drug put me in the Medicare donut hole, which meant I had to bear the full cost of all drugs until I reached the maximum out of pocket amount. Then I fell into the catastrophic category and was only required to pay a percentage of the cost of all drugs. Thankfully this was the only time that would happen during my treatment. The other good news was I found out that after two years on social security disability, I automatically qualified for Medicare even though I was not 65 years old.

In August I began four weeks of radiation, front and back and into the clavicle area. I tolerated this fairly well, even though I was warned, due to my very fair complexion, that I might burn severely and may have to delay some of the treatments. One thing I did have that surprised everyone was a series of very tiny blisters around the area of the radiation. Not in the field, just on the fringe of the radiated area. We finally determined that I was having an allergic reaction to the India ink that was used to mark the radiation field. So we switched to Magic Marker!

Sleeping was tricky during this time since both my front and back were burned. I slept on my side propped with pillows. I used straight aloe gel on the radiated area twice daily, even before any burning appeared.

There is some apprehension that goes along with radiation, like: What if I breathe too deeply? What if I sneeze or cough? Will the radiation shift and injure any organs? To clear my restless mind, I would mentally count starting with a really large number: 10,753, 10,754, 10,755, etc. I had to focus on the numerical sequence and couldn't focus on frightful things that may or may not happen.

Since the medical office where I worked was just across the street from the cancer center, I was able to work a light schedule during this time. I would report to work at 9:00 a.m., leave at 3:00 p.m. for my radiation, go home, take a nap, get up, fix dinner, and then go back to bed for the night...repeating the whole thing again the next day. I was told that a couple weeks into the treatment, it was quite common to hit a wall and get very fatigued. I never noticed this and just wanted all the treatment to be completed. I could see a light at the end of this nine-month tunnel.

The End of Treatments

On Labor Day weekend of 1998, we celebrated the end of my cancer treatments. There were many nights of sleeplessness, leg cramps, heel spurs, and chemo-induced arthralgia and a time when my blood counts went haywire. My cholesterol went to almost 500 and liver enzymes were extremely high with tumor markers elevated, spurring the decision to biopsy my liver. It was clear of any cancer (whew), but we didn't have an answer for the abnormal lab work. After much head scratching, being placed on cholesterol meds which wouldn't affect the liver, a liver ultrasound and biopsy, and changing to Femara, we finally tested my thyroid. It was extremely hyperactive. I was prescribed a thyroid suppressant for quite a few years and had intermittent ultrasounds. Early on one showed a couple of nodules that were also biopsied (also no cancer, yay!). We monitored my tumor markers, thyroid, liver, and cholesterol for several years, and then I made the decision to have my thyroid removed. I now take Synthroid every day and am doing fine. Tumor markers, liver enzymes, and cholesterol are all back in the normal ranges.

I have also been diagnosed with type II diabetes and take a pill for that. I am definitely 25-30 pounds heavier than I want to be, but don't have the energy or motivation to exercise or diet on a regular basis. I find that my old body just won't heal the way it used to. Chronic joint and muscle aches and pains are a part of my life, but I won't let that stop me from doing what I want to do. I worked full time and we were able to travel until the lymphedema became a more constant aggravation. I applied for and received disability payments from Social Security after appealing several decisions.

I have had no recurrence since my original treatment in 1998 and was doing great until January 2017, when I developed a really strange bacterial infection in my right chest wall (the mastectomy side), which progressed into cellulitis, hospitalization, IV antibiotics, and surgery. When the surgeon opened up my chest on March 30 to debride the infection, she discovered a large mass of necrotic tissue and very little bleeding. Part of a rib was removed and a part of the large semi-circle incision had difficulty healing. I was referred to an infectious disease doctor and prescribed a PICC line for IV antibiotics for 6 weeks, then oral antibiotics through September 2018. In addition, I had wound care several times a week, which included packing the underlying cavern in my chest and cleaning the open wound. The necrosis of tissue and bone was determined to have been caused by radiation treatment in 1998 to my front and back and clavicle areas. After many consultations, including a visit to the Mayo Clinic in Minnesota, the consensus of recommendations was for a chest resection surgery to remove three to four ribs, to cover the lung, and to transfer muscle from my back to my front to cover the wound.

I was petrified. The first surgery in March 2017, and I had considerable pain and wound care afterwards. Based on my consultation with the radiation therapy director, who told me, "It will heal—it will just take a very long time," I opted for hyperbaric therapy, which was suggested as a method of encouraging healing and was especially helpful for open wounds in diabetics. I obtained a referral from my doctor and endured thirty sessions and travelled 50 miles each way to try to get my chest to heal without further surgery. The wound was determined fully closed in April 2018, although I stayed on antibiotics until September

2019 to make sure all the bacteria were eliminated. Pathology determined the bacteria to be Simulans A, which is not very common and is resistant to many antibiotics. According to the infectious disease doctor, it often hibernates and reoccurs, so caution was advised. Plus, I was told that since not all the necrotic tissue was removed at the time of the first surgery, the necrosis may continue and flare up at a later date.

My insurance (PPO) would not allow me to go to M.D. Anderson, and it would not let me go on a private pay basis due to their agreement with Medicare! I had discovered that there was a long-term cancer survivor's group at M.D. Anderson, and when making my decisions, it would have been helpful to discuss my experience with others that may have had the same or similar thing happen. The local cancer centers, in my opinion, did not have a history of long- term survivors' complications or access to patients' histories after being determined NED.

Sadly, my brother was not so lucky. His lymphoma recurred four different times and he tried many new medications and experimental treatments through his caregivers at Johns Hopkins. He passed away in 2007.

My children and my husband's children have produced 11 grandchildren who we enjoy immensely. The online Erase IBC group was a lifesaver over the years with information on protocols and side effects...I know treatments are soooo different nowadays.

I lost my husband in 2016 to pulmonary fibrosis, but we had many wonderful years together. Today I feel good but wonder whether I will have to do this battle again or another cancer battle one of these days. In the meantime...I have many travel plans and I have informed my three grown children that when I run out of money, I'm moving in!

I am flattered to be asked to tell my story. Pray for all of us WARRIORS! New treatments and drugs are coming out every year. Those statistics that everyone wants to research and make sense of don't apply to us anymore. Keep up the good fight, sisters!

Pat (74 years young and experienced!)

Amy Pitman

Prayer, Laughter, and a Positive Attitude

Diagnosis

On January 2, 2002, at the age of 37, I was diagnosed with Inflammatory Breast Cancer (IBC). I was a single mom with a nine-year-old daughter, Mallory. The first thing I did was call my parents and my sister. We were all devastated, but we started researching this type of cancer. We all found out that IBC is a very aggressive and rare type of breast cancer and only about four percent of all breast cancer cases are IBC. I was told that only 40 percent of these cases survive more than five years. Right then, I decided that I was going to be in the 40 percent.

Family History

My family did have a history of cancer. My grandmother and two aunts had either ovarian cancer or inflammatory breast cancer, all at an early age, and two of them died before they were 41 years old. Due to this history, my doctors suggested that I have genetic testing. I tested positive for the BRCA2 breast cancer gene, as did my mom and sister.

Treatment and a Plan

Therefore, I decided to get a plan. I remembered what some teachers always told me: Form a plan, then work the plan. So, this is what I did. My doctors had a plan so I had to have one too. My doctors told me their plan of four rounds of chemo, then surgery, then four more rounds of chemo, then six weeks of daily radiation. My plan was prayer, laughter, and a positive attitude. I started praying and I asked for everyone's prayers. Then, my friends and family asked for all of their friends and families' prayers. I was on all types of churches prayer lists all over the nation. I did not believe God wanted me to die. Again, I believed God had a plan too!

I also knew that I had to be positive and hopeful. Even on my worst days after chemo, I knew I had to fight and be hopeful for my family, my friends, and my daughter. People were so amazed at my attitude that it gave them hope that I was not going to die.

But humor and laughter have always been a big part of my personality and laughter has gotten me through some other really tough times in my life. My daughter thought it was so much fun and so funny when she and her friends helped my friends shave my head. Also, since I was single, I still continued to go out with friends when I was feeling good. But, because I had no body hair then, I wore a bandana most days (never a wig – it was way too hot in Texas) and drew my eyebrows on with a brow pencil. My motto at the end of an evening out was, "You know you had a good time when your bandana is not on straight and you come home with only one eyebrow!"

God, my parents, sister, daughter, and friends were my driving forces. Medically, my body reacted very well with the chemo, surgery and radiation. Additionally, it was everyone's prayers, laughter, and positive attitude that helped me to survive.

Everyone including God worked their plan, and I am still alive after 18 years from diagnosis.

Positive Changes

Cancer changed my life! I actually took better care of myself. I have always been very active, but cancer made me be more aware of my diet, exercise, and knowledge that my life is precious. I was 37 when I was diagnosed and I thought I would live forever. Well, I won't, and now I live life to the fullest. I am very blessed to be very healthy now. I want to enjoy life more with my family and quality friends. I have lost many friends from cancer. I have gained more friends and have been able to help lots of other survivors. I, along with several other women, started a Young Survivors group in Fort Worth, Texas. We helped many women in their journeys. I would meet with or just talk to survivors and try to give them hope in their fight. I was very active in the breast cancer community, but now I help people on a one-on-one basis. I try to have a balanced life with family, friends, hobbies, church, work, and community service. I don't think you ever can "move on" from breast cancer. You just live your life a little differently.

Chin Up...tomorrow is a new day!

Rosemary Heise

I saw a sweatshirt that said: "I am not an alcoholic. I am a drunk. Alcoholics attend meetings." I think it was supposed to be funny. But who would want to admit being a drunk? This story is not about being an alcoholic, but alcohol plays a part in it. I had been living a non-life for years...no direction, no purpose, and certainly going nowhere. This story starts after a friend and I had been out—as we had been numerous times before. We tried to get together a couple times a month, talk very intelligently, speak with great humor and in general just be very entertaining. She drove that night, which was very unusual. Normally I did. On the way home, we were pulled over. That night, she got a DUI. That year, I got cancer. And so I start.

Symptoms and Diagnosis

Around Thanksgiving 1993, I visited the doctor because of a very warm, reddened breast. I was lucky. The doctor diagnosed it correctly right away. Many times, inflammatory breast cancer is diagnosed as mastitis and the correct treatment is delayed.

Treatment

I started chemotherapy after the first of the year in 1994, which was followed by surgery and radiation. My family was in shock but did not let me see their fears. My friends gathered around me, creating protection and a safe haven. I was stunned by the outpouring of love and prayers from complete strangers. I remember very little about the next few months. All I knew was that I had breast cancer and I was going to die. A friend gave me a book by Dr. Bernie Siegel called *Love, Medicine and Miracles*. When I read it, I felt like Dr. Siegel came out of the book and slapped me along side the head. He offered hope. I formulated a plan. Maybe I could live—even for a little while. I had to try.

Coping techniques

There were things I had to do to live. I prepared a list: Eat right and drink water, exercise, take supplements, find my creative self, meditate and pray...and play. I had to do them all if I were going to live. And so I started. But I quickly found out that that wasn't a good plan at all. I felt that if I didn't meditate for 20 minutes, I was going to die; if I ate something I wasn't supposed to, I was going to die. And play? I hadn't played for years— probably didn't even remember how. The stress of trying to live was going to do me in! Then I came across a solution to this problem. Focus on one thing at a time, the easiest one first. When that became automatic, go to the next.

I figured taking pills seemed to be the easiest way to start, so I started a rather by-guess-and-by-golly supplement plan. In 2000, I started working with a Doctor of Naturopathy for a more structured program. At one meeting with my cancer support group, I shared a dream I had had earlier. I dreamed I had died—I could feel it! It was so vivid—so real—so very frightening. Was it a premonition? One woman suggested that perhaps it represented a dying to my old self and being reborn as a new person. It was a very comforting thought. But I certainly didn't know it was scriptural. (Ephesians 4:22-23 says: "So get rid of your old self which made you live as you used to... your hearts and minds must be made completely new and you must put on the new self.")

Recurrence

In 1997, the cancer returned. Even though I was stronger than
I was in 1994, this was a very difficult time. Chemotherapy did
nothing. I temporarily moved to Rochester, MN, where I took
more radiation and ended up with bad radiation burns. The
radiation did not stop the cancer. The tumor was moving up
my neck, around my back and inching around my waist. I had
done some research and had found a hospital in Mexico that
offered alternatives to standard treatment. I felt I needed to
take a chance. It was a frightening idea, but I felt I had no choice
and decided to go. Before I left, a woman I didn't know at the
time asked me out to lunch. She gave me some books about
God to take with me. She offered to pray for me. Although I was
uncomfortable at the time, I was very touched and took the
material with me. I really didn't know much about having God in
my life. My God-life was limited to evening prayers.

At the hospital in Mexico, I met with other women and we
had daily prayers. I met a wonderful husband/wife couple who
also offered prayers. They gave me a copy of *My Daily Bread*, a
daily meditation booklet. I know at one point I prayed the prayer
of salvation, but I didn't feel differently. I was trying to get to
know God, but I was struggling.

After two separate trips to Mexico, I came home stronger
physically but with no plans for further treatment. There
wasn't anything. I was starting to lose hope. A friend had been
researching a new drug called Herceptin. It had not yet been
approved for use by the FDA. She tried to see if I could get it
through their compassionate-use program, but it was only
offered through lottery. However, it was due to be approved for
use in the fall of 1998.

Additional Treatment

On December 31, 1998, I had my first treatment of Herceptin. It
did not offer a cure, but it stopped the spread of the disease and
the existing tumor faded. I continued with my wellness program.
With proper supplements and eating right, I was feeling stronger
and more confident. I had a new puppy and was learning to play;

guided imagery tapes assisted me with meditation. I played only soothing music and excluded TV programs with violence. Finally, I started an exercise program. But where was God? I didn't get it. Where do I turn? Do I go back to church? I know my birth church had been praying for me and I had attended some services, but I didn't feel anything. Why was this so difficult?

My niece asked me to attend a service at her church. That Sunday was an experience that was certainly very different from anything I had had before. People seemed joyful; they seemed to feel that God was there in the church with them, and they were praising out loud. I was touched and moved to tears. After church I drove around, uncertain about my feelings over this new experience. I wanted more of this, but did it mean that I was to give up the church I was baptized in? I was crying and asking God for some message. The Christian radio station I had on in the car was playing music. All of a sudden it seemed like the tape got stuck or something and the words became a mass of garbled nonsense. I was stunned, and amid the tears, laughed out loud. It sounded like my idea of speaking in tongues! Yes, I was on the right path.

I started attending Grace Life in 2000. I know that when I did, I felt I was where I needed to be.

I have had many surgeries and treatments since December of 1998. The radiation treatments substantially damaged my chest wall and I was experiencing draining of fluid. I visited doctors to see what could be done, and we chose to try the hyperbaric chamber. In August of 2002, I started 11 weeks of daily trips to Sioux Falls, SD. The chamber didn't fix the problem, but it made it possible for me to have surgery. In January of 2003 I had reconstructive surgery. Tissue and muscle were taken from my back, and skin taken from my thighs was grafted to cover my chest. It was a painful experience, but it healed well and worked. Prior to the operation, I had asked the surgeon if he would remove my left breast at the same time. Its presence was a daily reminder that I could get cancer there too. The surgeon felt that two surgeries would have been too much and said it could be done at a later date.

A New Cancer

By April of 2003, I had developed a spot on the skin of my left breast, and a biopsy determined cancer. After a few unsuccessful chemo treatments, surgery was performed in May. When I removed the bandages during the healing process, I noticed that the surgeon did not remove the one area that had the tumor, so it was back to the surgeon for more work.

Another Cancer

In 2004, I noticed a couple spots on my back. I again visited the oncologist. The spots tested positive for cancer cells. I tried two other treatments unsuccessfully then had the surgeon remove the spots. Unfortunately, the after-surgery pathology report indicated the presence of cancer cells in one area, so I went back in again.

Treatment and Response

Between 2005 and approximately 2008, I started and ended treatments with Avastin (causing terrible bloody noses), Tykerb (causing serious diarrhea) and topical Aldara on my shoulder blade (causing open lesions) for a tumor on my right shoulder and in the clavicle region. In March of 2013 I added Kadcyla. It was very effective on cancer activity on left shoulder blade but did nothing for the right shoulder/clavicle mass. In March of 2014 I stopped Kadcyla and had 25 radiation treatments on my right shoulder. A cancerous lymph node appeared on the left side of my neck so I had that removed. I lost partial use of my arm and started physical therapy. An MRI and an Xray showed possible tumor activity in the left humerus bone. In August of 2014 I started Perjeta without the Taxotere.

A Life Philosophy

The county music singer Lari White says: "This ain't no stumblin' block, it's just a steppin' stone." Well each one of these little steppin' stones has made me stronger. As for the cancer that has chosen a home in my body, I must refuse to see recurrence as a failure. I must view it as a message. I need to understand the message and decide what my response will be. For me, the message of recurrence is clearly that I am not taking care of myself as I needed to. I have not been as careful in following the diet I knew was best for me. Only occasionally do I work with my creative self. And the big one: I have only partially resolved my emotional issues and I still deal with occasional bouts of sadness. I do know, however, that God has been and always is in my life. That is evidenced by times of joy and periods of wonderful health.

I have little cards around my house as comforters. One of my favorite and most often used is from II Corinthians 4:8: "We are often troubled, but not crushed; sometime in doubt, but never in despair. There are many enemies, but we are never without a friend; and though badly hurt at times, we are not destroyed." Also from II Corinthians 4:16: "So we're not giving up. How could we! Even though on the outside it often looks like things are falling apart on us, on the inside, where God is making new life, not a day goes by without His unfolding grace." And in closing, John Newton, the composer of "Amazing Grace," said in *The Christian Pioneer*: "Though I am not what I ought to be, nor what I wish to be, nor what I hope to be, I can truly say, I am not what I once was;...By the Grace of God, I am what I am."[165]

---

165 Rosemary Heise lost her battle with IBC on April 15, 2016, after living with IBC for 23 years. She was 68 years old.

Jeannine Donahue

In 2007, 29 days before my 27th birthday, I underwent a double mastectomy. Six months prior I was told, after being previously misdiagnosed, that I had a rare and extremely aggressive form of cancer called inflammatory breast cancer, also known as IBC. I had a late stage cancer that accounted for under five percent of all breast cancers, and it was a disease that lacked statistics and had hardly any research.

Diagnosis

My journey started when I noticed my left breast was slightly swollen with a rash and I was having sharp shooting pains. After going to my gynecologist, I was told I had a mammary duct infection and was given an antibiotic. In the meantime, I found a lump in my armpit that was missed initially. I learned later this was a swollen lymph node. Because there was no improvement, I had a needle biopsy, which showed I had ductal carcinoma in situ, or DCIS—the most common type of non-invasive breast cancer. I had hoped that my worries would be quickly resolved with a surgical procedure. Little did I know that everything was about to get worse.

The breast surgeon I was referred to suggested an immediate single mastectomy but refused any other procedure on the rash. So I was sent off to see a plastic surgeon. At the plastic surgery consultation, the doctor stated he wouldn't operate on me until the rash was looked at. I didn't know it at the time, but that plastic surgeon saved my life.

He referred me to another breast surgeon for a second opinion. That surgeon spoke to my parents and me for the first time about a different type of breast cancer, one that didn't require the presence of a lump. In fact, all the symptoms I had—breast swelling, sharp shooting pain, a rash—were all signs of inflammatory breast cancer. Unlike DCIS, IBC needs to be treated with preoperative systemic chemotherapy to help shrink the tumor, then a mastectomy, followed by radiotherapy.

I was speechless. Here I was, a young adult with no family history of breast cancer and no signs of the typical gene mutations associated with breast cancer, BRCA 1 and BRCA 2. Yet, I was diagnosed with late-stage inflammatory breast cancer. Without treatment, I was told I had six months to live. With treatment, my prognosis was also quite poor—likely only a few years.

I felt almost hopeless, but I was determined to take my chances.

Treatment

For six years, I underwent treatment for IBC. Treatment was grueling. After chemotherapy, I was bald, with gray skin. All the surgeries left me feeling like I had been taken apart and pieced back together again. Radiation was exhausting and left me burnt to a crisp. Looking at myself in the mirror was like looking at my own corpse. Cancer stripped me of everything I knew. While I recognized that I was lucky to be alive, I also mourned the person I was before IBC entered my vocabulary and I realized that that mentally— facing my own mortality—I would carry with me for the rest of my life.

Advocacy

Now, 13 years after my initial diagnosis, I am healthy and I can proudly state that I have no evidence of disease.

Surviving IBC put me on a new path, one of advocacy that would include stops on Capitol Hill to lobby for more research. It also led me to a physician who would become my mentor—and boss. I now help run the Precision Medicine program at Northwestern University in Chicago, under my former IBC doctor, now boss, Dr. Massimo Cristofanilli. Our team of health care providers, researchers, and scientists focus on the uniqueness of each person and their cancer to provide a tailored treatment plan for each person. Through my work with other late stage cancer patients, I have found a way to continue my fight against cancer. To me research and precision medicine go hand in hand and are vital components in the fight against cancer.

This is just my story, my journey with a disease that even now, 13 years later, lacks enough research, and I lack understanding of why I not only got IBC, but survived when so many others have not.

We all have been touched in one way or another by an untreatable disease. It is a helpless, and at times, hopeless place to be. We have all asked "Why" and "How" and "What can I do?" I stand here as proof of three things: there is always hope, there is always a way to fight, and research is vital for both!

Together we stand here almost 50 years after the signing of the National Cancer Act of 1971 that pushed for increased research in an effort to find a cure. Though we have come very far in our knowledge, we still have a great deal to learn. This is due to the fact that we are each so extraordinarily unique, which in turn makes our disease unique as well.

Going Forward

No two cancer patients are the same. We could each carry the same diagnosis but how our cancer grows, why it grows, where it grows, and the rate at which it grows can be vastly different. This difference stems from many factors, which include: our genetics (what we get from our parents), our genomics (how the genes in our body live and interact with each other), and our epigenetics (how the outside world affects us on a cellular level).

With all of these factors you have a uniqueness as vast as the human race.

I graduated college with a degree in Accounting, but I joke that I also have PhD in cancer. I learned the language and the culture and I became an advocate for myself. When my treatment ended I became an advocate for those who have been taken from this earth as a result of cancer, and for those who unfortunately will one day face the journey of a cancer diagnosis.

So why am I telling you all of this? Because within each of us we hold a story, individually unique, but when combined and compared, could have the power to become a tool in the prevention, detection, and treatment of disease. Not only do our voices have power, so do our genes. They are our unique blueprint. This blueprint holds in it the data that documents how we are designed.

I am sounding a call to action—let us unite our blueprints to build a solid foundation of research that can be used to create a more precise, effective and efficient way to detect, prevent, and treat disease. Let us learn from one another to create a path to better health for all!

To quote Helen Keller, "Alone we can do so little; together we can do so much."

Vanetta Harrington

I have been a breast cancer survivor since 1992.

Earlier cancer treatment

My cancer started with the left breast. I had been told by my primary care doctor to have frequent mammograms because my breasts were dense and large, which made it difficult to do breast exams.

In 1992 the mammogram results showed a lump on the left breast. I had a lumpectomy, and fortunately did not have any medication such as radiation or chemotherapy.

I did well for the next two and one half years with no problems until August of 1994. I had a mammogram that showed calcification in the right breast. Again the doctor performed a lumpectomy as he did on the left breast in 1992.

Diagnosis of IBC

I thought everything was going along fine until 1997, when I was diagnosed with inflammatory breast cancer. Less than 4 percent of women who get this type survive it, although with newer drugs, women are living longer.

Treatment of IBC

As part of my treatment for inflammatory breast cancer I was given a stem cell transplant. I spent several days in the hospital. My husband and family were very supportive during this time. Our youngest son, Brandon, was only five years old and developed chicken pox and could no longer come to the hospital for visits.

Other Cancers

While I was fighting inflammatory breast cancer, I learned in 1998 that a malignant neoplasm had formed on my scalp and was not related to my breast cancer. The doctor did a re-excision on this area.

Going Forward

Today, I am feeling fine. However a few years back I was diagnosed with a brain tumor. I had surgery and radiation. So far God has been fantastic. I am so grateful that he has taken me under his wing. Now it is 2018 and I have been told that I have a tumor near the pancreas. I am on a pill form of chemotherapy and have had no side-effects, and the tumor is shrinking.

I wanted you to know that cancer is not always a death sentence. Put your trust in the Lord!!!!

If he did it before he can do it again.

Remember get your mammograms!!!!!!!!!

Anne K. Abate, Ph.D.
My IBC Story

I have learned many things in the last few years. These are things that I hope nobody else ever has to learn. While I am a strong proponent of continuing education for everyone, you will see why I do not want anyone to follow my path.

Symptoms

I had odd symptoms for almost a year before I was actually diagnosed. One breast was extremely itchy—all the time. It also started to swell and turn very red. In addition, I would often break out in small patches of rash on various parts of my body—hands, arms, face, legs—a different place each time, and then they would suddenly and mysteriously just go away. Although a smart, educated woman, I was a medical idiot. I did not go to the doctor, nor even schedule a mammogram. I was only 43 years old, after all, and not ready for this to happen. But, I was a librarian, so I researched everything online. This was 2001 and the Internet was already a scary place. I saw many images of breast cancer and practically diagnosed myself. I finally decided to go straight to a breast surgeon, since I was convinced of my self-diagnosis. I called the local breast center and asked for an appointment. They asked me which doctor I wanted to see and I asked them to name all of them. It is strange to believe, but I selected my surgeon because she had the same name as a brand of wine we enjoy!

Diagnosis

In February of 2002—February 14 to be exact—I was diagnosed with an aggressive disease known as inflammatory breast cancer. This is not your regular "plain vanilla" breast cancer, and it should not be treated in the same way. Within a week of the original diagnosis, I had undergone two surgeries—the first two surgeries of my life—one to do an extensive biopsy and the other to insert a subdermal port in my upper chest through which I would receive chemotherapy for the next six months.

Treatment

Chemotherapy is hard—very hard. After all, they are trying to kill off actively dividing cells in your body. Eating is impossible. You never sleep because of the steroids they give you to make you try to feel normal. I am proud to say that I did work full time throughout those treatments and only missed work on the days of treatment. On those days, which at that time would occur every three weeks, you receive massive doses of the poison. My special day occurred every third Friday. After treatment, I would go out to lunch with friends. You do not really feel bad until the third day after treatment, so on treatment days, I was at my best and could enjoy a good lunch.

In August, I went under the knife again, this time for a bilateral mastectomy. For me, the surgery was easy. You just go to sleep and when you awake, it is all over, and various parts of your body are gone. I was determined to not lose range of motion in my arms which often happens after breast surgery, so I actually started exercising in the hospital bed on the afternoon of the surgery.

My medical team finished everything off with a few weeks of radiation in the fall of that year. Radiation is really the scariest part of the entire process. They put you in this room completely encased in three feet of concrete. Everyone else scurries out of the room before they shoot beams of skin-killing light at you.

I did not realize that the treatments would also cause loss of appetite and other odd symptoms. And to skip forward 15 years, radiation treatments can also cause long-term changes to the skin. The gift that keeps on giving!

I am happy to say that after the surgery, I was declared cancer-free. In just a few months after my active treatment ended, some of my strength started to return, and I was almost back to normal.

Advocacy

Following my treatment, and even while I was in treatment, I became more active in advocacy groups and support organizations. I discovered the Inflammatory Breast Cancer Research Foundation and become active in their efforts to educate the world about this terrible form of cancer. I also became a volunteer in the Reach to Recovery Program of the American Cancer Society. Through this program, breast cancer survivors reach out to newly diagnosed patients to offer them support, an ear, and a path forward. That program now has an online component where patients can chat online with survivors. At the same time, I have become more active in the American Cancer Society through the years and was the co-lead on the National Volunteer Training Team. I was recently selected to be a Stakeholder for the American Cancer Society Extramural Research Department that reviews grants that are sponsored by ACS.

Several years ago, I learned about the Department of Defense Breast Cancer Research Program and the role of the Consumer Reviewer. I jumped at the opportunity to use my fairly well-trained academic abilities to read and think and write, to combine those with my personal experiences with an awful disease and the side effects of treatment, and to discover this tremendous way to really make a difference to the future of medical research. I was delighted when one of my staff partners at the American Cancer Society agreed to sponsor me as a Consumer Reviewer.

About 10 years ago, I started volunteering at my local breast center. Every week, I see literally hundreds of women sitting in the waiting room in little pink vests waiting for their mammograms. Each week, dozens of these women will be diagnosed with breast cancer. We all need to work together to stop this nonsense.

A New Treatment

Several years ago, my wonderful oncologist and his team recommended adding a brand new drug called Ibrance to the mix of things we were using at the time to ward off any progression of my disease. In my research of this new drug, I discovered that it was just released to the market, having been pulled out of clinical trial early. I was thrilled to find out that some of the initial research on this drug had been supported under the Department of Defense Breast Cancer Research Program. What an amazing thing to know that I am helping advance research that could actually be helping me to stay alive. I now have even more reasons to be involved in these research programs.

In the last few years, I have had too many scans and tests and biopsies to count. I have experienced scares and flare-ups of my disease over the years, but up until recently, my medical team has been able to fight those back and keep active disease away from me. Several years ago, I was diagnosed as having active metastatic disease, but I certainly did not know where it was hiding at the time. Then, in mid-2019, I ended up in intensive care for a full week. I could barely breathe and was experiencing pain that I thought was from breaking a rib several years ago. After many more tests and exploration, they diagnosed metastatic disease in my abdomen, liver, bones, and perhaps spine and skull. This meant I was back in active treatment and will remain on some sort of treatment for the rest of my life. My current cocktail includes a rather new drug called Verzenio. That is given along with Faslodex and Zometa, and usually fluids. Now my treatments are once every four weeks. I always jump at the opportunity to try the latest and greatest drugs and treatments.

I am hoping that they will continue to develop these novel therapies that will be able to keep me alive for a very long time.

Lessons Learned

My experiences have taught me some very important lessons.

First, life is too short. Simply that. Life is too short. It is important to do everything that you can in the time that you have.

Next, I have developed an astounding ability to say and do what needs to be said and done. I have always been pretty vocal. Now I realize how important that is and plan to speak up whenever necessary. I am no longer afraid to say anything or ask anything. This has served me well in my roles as a Consumer Reviewer and ACS Stakeholder. I am there to speak the words of the breast cancer patient and survivor in order to help improve treatment and reduce side effects, and some day stop this madness that is breast cancer.

Take care of yourself. I would encourage you to learn a little bit about inflammatory breast cancer for yourselves and for the women you know. The motto of the Inflammatory Breast Cancer Research Foundation is "You don't have to have a lump to have breast cancer," and this is really true. The symptoms are entirely different from that plain vanilla breast cancer. I encourage you to go to www.ibcresearch.org and learn the symptoms. There are brochures and bookmarks that you can print out and share with others.

Do not learn things the hard way—the way I did. Continuing education is essential, but none of us need to know as much as I do about chemotherapy and surgical procedures and radiation treatments and hormonal therapies. Fortunately, within the education I have had over the last twenty years, I did learn that first most important lesson: life is short—make sure you use it, every minute of it, wisely.

Kim Alexander

Warrior. That's the term used in the cancer community to describe a person who has survived the initial diagnosis and adjuvant treatment and who continues treatment. And a term I never in a million years believed would be used to describe me.

Yet, here I am on what is soon to be the 14th anniversary of my diagnosis of IBC.[166] A day does not go by that I don't think about that horrible time in my life, nor does a day go by that I don't feel incredibly humbled to still be here and actually living the life I have always dreamed of living. It's a quiet life, filled with the tranquility of the company of my dogs, my 23-year-old cat and three thoroughbred horses, all ex-racehorses. I have never been one to want much. But this is everything to me. It's as if I was literally born again.

Unlike so many, I have been extremely fortunate in that I don't have to cope with some pretty severe side effects that many have been burdened with in the aftermath of their treatments. This is not to say I don't have them, but only to say that they are not encroaching on my day-to-day life, nor minimizing my ability to enjoy the past few years.

---

166 Kim's original diagnosis is discussed in *Nobody's Listening,* a collection of patient stories published in 2014.

IBC Returns

There was a rough patch after my initial treatments.[167] Five months after finishing the standard protocol, including a two-year regimen of Herceptin, I discovered a swelling on my non-cancer side, the left side, which a biopsy revealed to be IBC, albeit with a pathology that was somewhat different from the first one. Unfortunately, nobody can accurately determine whether this was a progression of my disease, a recurrence, or even a new cancer altogether, as I had not had any scans other than the one for the initial diagnosis. This oversight could have proved very problematic or even deadly for me; however, I guess I lucked out. At that point I entered into numerous treatments, some standard, some clinical trials—none of which were able to completely remove the tumors that remained local to my left breast, chest wall and lymph nodes (and a questionable spot or two on my liver). They were successful in reducing the burden of disease, yet NED (no evidence of disease) was still elusive for me. The treatments were rapid-fire and the toxicity from all those chemicals had me reduced to what I would liken to a zombie of sorts with my quality of life becoming unacceptable. I had, in fact, decided to call it quits.

However, in December of 2010 I found my way to Sarah Cannon Cancer Center in Nashville in a last attempt to find a treatment that would work—or at least buy me some time with an acceptable quality of life. There, I was placed in the capable hands of Dr. Denise Yardley, who had a space for me in a clinical trial for a drug then known as TDM-1, and later, after it's approval from the FDA, known as Kadcyla. (I gave it the moniker "Godzilla.") After enough time was allowed to let the other treatments wash out of my system, I began the trial.

Response to the New Treatment

It was a game-changer for me. Better put, a lifesaver. Almost immediately scans began showing the tumors shrinking and by

---

167 Kim's initial treatment was Adriamycin and Cytoxan—four doses every two weeks, then weekly doses of Taxol and Herceptin for 12 weeks. This was followed by surgery and then radiation.

December of 2011, I was waiting in the room for scan results—which had become very routine yet no less terrifying—when Dr. Yardley walked into the room and asked me how I was. I thought that was kind of an odd question to ask ME when SHE was the one with the scan results in her hands. I said, "I don't know, how am I?" She quietly replied with a stone cold poker face, "Well, I don't know. The scan results here only have one sentence... hmmmm, let me see...Oh, yeah...'Scans show no evidence of active disease in this patient.'" Then she just looked at me. I was NOT expecting THAT. Humorously, during the year that I had spent with these lovely and caring folks at Sarah Cannon/Tennessee Oncology, they had never heard me use a curse word. But at that moment, as I looked into my teary-eyed doctor, my only response was, "You're shitting me."

We still laugh about that moment. And I am still NED. Warrior. Survivor. Thriver.

Call me whatever you like. I am fortunate in every way imaginable. Blessed beyond my wildest belief. While I am still getting Herceptin infusions once a month, it is considered "preventive" and...knock wood...it has been working.

There's an old saying that goes, "If I'd have known I was going to live this long, I would have taken better care of myself."

While we all appreciate the humor in that comment, there is a profound truth to it as well. In hindsight, I realize there were many mistakes made by my first oncologist and also by my second one. Yes, I switched. And to this day I believe that had I stayed the course with my first doctor, I might not be here. The change is a hard one to make. We all want to believe our oncologist is going to be our salvation. We tend to place them high in lofty esteem, as though they are more like a sort of god than a flawed human being. Yet, even the best-intentioned doctor is still capable of making mistakes—mistakes, in this setting, that can cost us our lives. The third time was, thankfully, a charm as well as a lifesaver.

Looking Ahead

If I were to offer any advice to newbies, I would say most definitely arm yourself with as much information as you can, ask a TON of questions, take copious notes, and, hopefully, have a person who can be an advocate and a voice for you when your own rational thoughts are elusive. NEVER be afraid to seek other opinions and, if you must, change doctors. That, and just LIVE, because no matter how much time we have, it won't ever be enough.

Jenee Bobbora

My story is unusual and common at the same time. It depends on which view a person sees it through. Being diagnosed with inflammatory breast cancer at the age of 32 was certainly a shock. I knew people whose moms and grandmoms had been diagnosed with breast cancer, but being diagnosed at 32 was unheard of in my world. Once I crossed that invisible plane into the "breast cancer world," I realized my situation was pretty common: there are many other young women with breast cancer. Once you have the disease, you are welcomed into a new world full of strong and courageous people who have been through it before you.

Symptoms

I noticed some unusual symptoms in my breast; it was swollen and very painful. I went to see my OB/GYN to ask his opinion. He thought that the swelling was tied to the new birth control pill I had just begun a month earlier and tried to send me on my way. I pushed for a mammogram, but he refused and insulted my intelligence because I asked for one. He did me a favor—he made me mad. By the grace of God, the following week I saw another doctor, who thought I had an infection and prescribed Cipro, but as I was leaving the office he said, "If it's not better in a week, come in for a biopsy. There is a small chance it could be inflammatory breast cancer."

Diagnosis

A week went by but my symptoms worsened. The words "inflammatory breast cancer" were in the back of my mind and, more importantly, they were in the backs of my family's minds, so they pushed for me to go to The University of Texas MD Anderson Cancer Center for an exam. I did, and I found out not only that I did have inflammatory breast cancer but also that it had spread to the lymph nodes in my axilla and supraclavicular area. Because of the supraclavicular area involvement, I was originally told I was stage 4. This was later changed to 3c. After the diagnosis, I sat there with my husband, just shaking my head in disbelief, but also with a feeling of confidence I would not succumb to this. I believe that was God's Grace and I think it was key to my survival that I never allowed myself to think I might die.

Treatment

I had chemotherapy first, then surgery, then twice-a-day radiation therapy, then tamoxifen for ten years. The year 2003 was a long year, but I was onboard and subscribed to it all. The Big Hammer Theory (find the biggest hammer and use it NOW) was right up my alley. I wanted the doctors to give me all that they thought I could handle and then a little more, and I believe they did.

Coping Techniques

In my opinion, the worst thing about being diagnosed with breast cancer at a young age is the implication that you could die young and not have the chance to raise your children. The one thing that I am most grateful for is that I am here to raise my daughter, because I know with absolute certainty that no one on earth could possibly love her as much as I do, and I think she deserves to feel that love for as long as possible. My daughter was 2 when I was diagnosed, so dying for me was not an option. I say that as emphatically as I possibly can, knowing that somewhere deep inside me is the realization that life is not fair and just because you are emphatic about something doesn't make it so. Nevertheless, I told myself on a daily basis that I would survive, and when you combine that with the best cancer treatment in the world, it worked for me.

A Community of Support Groups

During my many doctor appointments and support group meetings, I met some really wonderful women. Most of them were at least 15 years older than me; many of them were 30 and 40 years older than me. All of them impressed me. Many of them became like mentors to me; they became people who I look up to and aspire to be like. I learned a lot of lessons being the young woman in the group, but the one thing we never had in common was the "kid factor." All of their children were grown, had been given a solid foundation, and were starting their own lives. Often I would miss out on activities with these women because I didn't want to be away from my daughter.

Slowly but surely, I started to meet other young women, some even younger than me, through a young survivors organization. This was a great place for us to meet and discuss our feelings and fears. When I was with these younger women, our main topics of conversation were the problems we were having with hormones, children, and fertility issues. Some had gone into menopause way too early because of chemotherapy; some had been advised to put themselves into menopause with surgery; and others worried about whether they would be able to have children after cancer treatment. I always wanted to have more children, but I would be 38 when I finished my 5-year tamoxifen treatment. Thirty-eight years old before I could even think about getting pregnant again. I ultimately chose to forgo another pregnancy in favor of longer tamoxifen treatment. I have such empathy for my friends who were diagnosed before they had their first child; for them, starting a family is suddenly a major life decision involving doctors, tests, risk, and worry.

When I was 32, I hardly even knew what estrogen was, much less what it was like to live without it. During treatment, I went into temporary menopause and experienced a glimpse of the hot flashes and other side effects before my ovaries suddenly started working again. I've witnessed many of my friends suffer the effects of early menopause long before they should have. I don't think enough is known about young women with breast cancer and about just how hard it is to "just have your ovaries taken out," as a few doctors have told me.

At about year 7, I took a break from my heavy involvement in my young survivors group. I have many excuses for doing so, but I know deep down that the real reason is that I wasn't sure how many more deaths I could handle. Our group has lost way too many women, all before age 40: a 23-year-old newlywed; a 27-year-old with a 2-year-old child; a 34-year-old with a 4-year-old child; and a 38-year-old who fought for 5 years and was never able to start a family. I could go on and on with these horror stories. It's just heartbreaking to see husbands at the funerals holding little children they have to raise alone. It's just not right. I also turned my attention to the small foundation I'd co-founded with Patti Bradfield, whose daughter Tina passed away from IBC, and Dr. Massimo Cristofanilli, who famously took an interest in IBC early in his career and is a leading expert and founder of the first IBC Clinic. Through EraseIBC.org, we help educate about the disease, an issue very near and dear to our hearts because we know so many women who were misdiagnosed due to the unusual presentation of IBC, many women who were not diagnosed until stage 4 because of early misdiagnosis and the fact that IBC metastasizes so quickly.

Going Forward

I have been fortunate to be completely cancer free for 17 years now; I believe that I am cured. I took the drug tamoxifen for a total of 10 years over a 12-year span. This was the subject of a lot of arguing with my own doctors, which was troubling to me at times because I do believe they are the best in the world.

Around year five of my tamoxifen treatment, the new aromatase inhibitors became the more popular drug. Study after study was suggesting that they were more effective than tamoxifen, but there was a major asterisk for me in these studies because they had all been done on post-menopausal women. I was not post-menopausal, since I was only 38 years old, and I would have been required to shut down my ovaries or have them removed in order to take the aromatase inhibitors. I did not want to put myself into menopause as I knew too well the side effects that many of my friends in support groups were having due to early menopause. Things like severe vaginal dryness, bone loss, brain fog, to name a few, did not seem to be a fair trade-off for a few percentage points off the chance of recurrence that had been shown in post-menopausal women. I dug into research at the MD Anderson library and found that in Europe, the ATLAS trial had been testing Adjuvant Tamoxifen Longer Against Shorter, looking at whether 10 years of tamoxifen would decrease recurrence more than 5 years would. I dug deep and I reached out to the people in charge of the trial in London, I got their updates and I read all the reports. My doctors told me they really did not like the way the study was designed and that they didn't feel it would ever produce the relevant data needed. I also read studies about the side effects of early menopause, many of which were discovered somewhat by accident by a doctor in California who saw a huge trend in illness of the women who had their ovaries removed, even at a later age. My case is a bit more complex than most because of my BRCA2 mutation, which tends to make everyone think you should just have every risk factor removed. There has to be a better way than shutting down the ovaries and then taking a drug that aims to block every trace of estrogen from the body, causing tons of side effects. I have often joked with my doctors, "I'm 39, I can't have any more children, and I have no breasts. Would you MIND if I kept my ovaries for a few more years?"

The problem with treating cancer of course is that you very often have to trade one side effect for the other and I understood that and was willing to accept the downside if there was enough of an upside. Because I had very few terrible side effects from tamoxifen and because I was feeling very intuitive about it being the correct drug for me, I pushed back against my doctor's advice. She reluctantly agreed to let me keep taking the tamoxifen while cautioning me about the rare but serious side effects of tamoxifen like uterine cancer and blood clots.

I was only seeing the doctor twice a year at this point, and each time I would come in with my latest research. I even had to write a letter to the tumor board to explain my case to them to get them to keep prescribing it. At year seven, they told me they would no longer prescribe the drug for me. At this point, I was somewhat okay with their decision. I felt I had probably pushed them to their limit and that I had achieved what I wanted, which was to extend out at age 40 when I knew it was less likely I was raging with estrogen. We had a great discussion about all the treatment I'd received, the best of the best, 72-hour infusion of "the red devil," aggressive removal of nearly all my breast tissue, and then super-aggressive tailor-made twice-a-day radiation. My doctor was correct in stating I had truly received the most aggressive cutting edge treatment possible. I loved my team and I knew they loved me. So I stopped the drug.

About a year and a half later I was having my morning coffee and watching a news story about the very important news coming out of the world-famous San Antonio Breast Cancer Conference and across the bottom of the screen the new ticker read: "ATLAS trial shows Tamoxifen, 10 years is better than 5." Huh?—I just sort of paused for a moment scratching my head and thinking, well the Europeans think that, but my docs didn't like the study. Within seconds the news ticker read: "MD Anderson believes this is an important revelation that can help lower recurrence rates." I was speechless, I was a little angry, and I was a little tickled to know that my instincts were so correct despite having zero medical training. I picked up the phone and let my wonderful PA know I would be expecting a prescription called in that day and I would go back on the drug and take it until I completed 10 years. I think they thought I was nuts, but darn it, I had a VERY strong gut feeling about this and so I did it. I appreciate so much that they listened to me. I believe to this day that my doctor's belief in me and desire for me to be cured was a huge factor in my survival.

Here I am 17 years later. Did taking tamoxifen over 12 years matter? Is that why my IBC will never recur? Was it worth the weight gain and the achiness I believe are attributed to tamoxifen? We will never know, but sometimes you just have to follow your heart and your gut.

When I was being treated, I chose to have a double mastectomy originally under the layman's theory that if you have cancer in one breast at age 32, the other breast is likely to have a problem one day. Then it turned out I tested positive for the BRCA2 mutation and that my "good breast" had lots of ductal carcinoma in situ, so I was even more sure that having a double mastectomy was the right choice for me. Having no breasts takes some getting used to, especially as I entered my late 30s and early 40s. Suddenly, all my friends are in this "sexy" phase where everyone is showing cleavage. Cleavage is the "new black," and I have none—I can't even fake it! On most days, it doesn't bother me too much, but when trying on new clothes or bathing suits I can get pretty depressed. The prosthesis only looks good in certain things. I am eligible for reconstruction, but it's going to be a long, difficult surgery, and I am just too busy for that. I am fortunate that my husband has made this a non-issue. I don't know how he's done it, but he has, and it has made my life so much easier and more carefree.

My marriage was profoundly positively affected by my diagnosis. The humility that comes with your husband helping you with drains or trying to keep a sterile area when dressing a CVC catheter is intense. My husband has been an absolute rock. I'm pretty sure God knew my life was going to be a bit of a volcano when he put him in my path. We can now laugh about the "in sickness and in health" part of our marriage vows because neither of us really believed we'd have to live up to those words until we were in our late 80s. When you're in your 30s, you are going and blowing and finding your way and trying to make a name for yourself. You aren't really established in anything, and with a diagnosis like this you have to take a few steps back. While I remain super grateful and try to maintain an attitude of gratitude, all that treatment and the subsequent constant worry in the back of my mind definitely took its toll in many areas of my life. I believe the BRCA2 mutation and the screening and added risk that goes along with that are also part of the cause of the brain fog, which I can often feel. Its pretty daunting when you sit down and look at all that BRCA2 puts you at increased risk for. Even so, I am happy I know about my mutation. Over the last 17 years, I found myself overweight and not looking so good much of the time which bothered me at some level but also just caused me to say "oh well, at least I am here" on most days. The further I get away from that day in March 2003, the better I look and feel. I just turned 50 and I probably look better and more vibrant that I did at 33, bloated, exhausted, anemic and fighting those recurrence demons with every ounce of my being.

I have found many positive things about having breast cancer at a young age. Mainly, I feel that the treatment wasn't as hard for me, that my body could "take it" better than an older person might have. I also feel that the fact that I was young and caring for a child who kept me very busy was a blessing. I was often way too busy to worry about cancer. On the surface I didn't think about it much; I didn't have the time to. However, I now can see in hindsight I was fighting a battle inside my brain. But, of course, there is always the perspective that one gains when facing a life-threatening illness.

My immediate friends are not cancer survivors. I like it that the people I see daily are not survivors because I know that on some level they have no idea what I went through, and I think I like that. If they knew, I think they'd treat me differently, and I feel different enough already. Sure, I snicker sometimes at their lists of huge problems that often involve the most trivial things, but I like it that they share them with me. I feel sometimes that I lack motivation or any semblance of an ego; I feel like it was almost beaten out of me. Sometimes, I get mad at myself and my lack of drive to get things done, but when I sit quietly I can come to an understanding internally that it is my breast cancer experience, and the large part of my brain that is occupied by a deep-seated worry that keeps me from being totally energized. I am working on releasing that, but it's been hard. I must say, I am getting a bit cocky now about my survival now; I feel sometimes like saying to cancer, "Take that, LOSER!," like I have won a contest or something.

Finally, to look at positives, which is what I preach and what I truly believe to be an important factor in surviving any disease, I can say that being young and having cancer can be seen as an opportunity because so many of the great experiences of my life have been due to having breast cancer. It has shaped me into a better person. I have to mention how blessed I was with my surrounding family. My mom and dad, as well as my in-laws, were incredibly supportive. Not all people are that lucky and it is my hope that those who don't have supportive family seek and get support elsewhere because you definitely need support to get through this. My parents helped with everything my husband, daughter and I needed and that took a lot of worry off of me. Getting to know doctors as friends and getting involved in advocacy work and fund-raising and being able to support other women has been very fulfilling for me. On many levels, this has all been a blessing to me and my family, but I have not yet reached the point where I can say, "I wouldn't trade it." If you ask me when I am 80, I will certainly say that I wouldn't trade it, but that's too much of a gamble now. I want to live a long, long life. I hope that my story can show people that there is light at the end of the tunnel. Having just turned 50, I can honestly say my life is better than ever. I am still involved with EraseIBC.org doing advocacy work and I love speaking to and supporting women and families all over the world. I am still involved with my beloved MD Anderson and have been featured in their advertising campaign. People reach out to me on social media when they read my story and I know that often they just want to know if I am still alive because that brings them hope. I'm always honored to respond and encourage them, it is more of a blessing to me than it is to them.

Amy Berman

Living Your Best Life with Inflammatory Breast Cancer

It's hard to imagine that people can live well in the face of cancer. I remember when I was first diagnosed with inflammatory breast cancer in 2010. I thought my life was over. I imagined that I would have a short and very difficult life. But thankfully, that wasn't the case.

My good life wasn't a matter of luck. It was because of the extra support I received from a group of health professionals known as a palliative care team. I'll explain more about this extra layer of support that goes along with the regular care and treatment from the oncologist. But first, here's my story.

Symptoms

I woke up one morning and noticed a small, strange looking red spot on my right breast, around the size of a dime. The skin was red and puckered like the skin of an orange. It just appeared out of the blue and I knew it just didn't look right. By some strange circumstance I had read an article on inflammatory breast cancer the previous month. The article talked about "peau d'orange" or skin of an orange as a possible sign of the disease. The article also said that inflammatory breast cancer had the worst outcomes of any form of breast cancer and that there was no cure.

I can imagine some people would give it time to see if the spot went away but not me. I called my primary care doctor and she fit me in that same day. My heart was in my mouth. I was so hoping to be wrong. But deep down, I knew.

The primary care doctor and nurse practitioner saw me together. As I opened the paper gown their faces changed. I saw concern and sadness. Their faces now mirrored mine. My doctor called an oncologist in front of me asked if she could get me fit in for a mammogram later that day. It was comforting to have people fit me in.

I kept thinking about the article. It said that inflammatory breast cancer is usually diagnosed as stage three or four, spread beyond the point of origin (the breast) or spread widely in the body. Maybe that wouldn't be the case for me. It just appeared and I was seeing the doctor, getting a mammogram. Maybe I would be that person who did everything right and got it in time.

I sat in a white robe waiting for the mammogram. There were five women waiting with me in a row of seats against the wall in a hallway. Outwardly, we looked like women at a spa waiting for our massage or maybe a mani-pedi. One by one, the women were called into the room at the end of the hall, then reseated in the hallway again as they checked the quality of the images. Some were called back to retake images.

They called my name. I could feel my own heartbeat. As the technician positioned me for the mammogram I told her to take the extra images. She looked at me sideways and chose not to respond. I'm sure she thought I was just nervous. But as she started the machine and looked at her screen, her eyes widened. It was like seeing my primary care doctor's face. We were there for a while. I guess she took the extra images.

Diagnosis

In the hallway once again with my spa buddies, I noticed the doctors and fellows—the oncology trainees—pouring into a tiny dark room directly across from where we were seated. The woman to my left was getting anxious. She thought they were looking at her mammogram. I knew it must be mine.

Inflammatory breast cancer is rare, only 1 to 2 percent of breast cancer cases. I stood up and went into the little room and said my name. I asked if they were my images. The radiologist asked the other people crammed into to the room to leave. She said, "Would you like to meet the enemy?" She guided me through everything on the screen.

The steps that followed in the coming days were a biopsy, which confirmed the disease, and a scan which showed the cancer had spread to my lower spine. That meant that I was stage 4. It was strange because I didn't feel sick but I had advanced cancer, an incurable and life-limiting disease. The National Cancer Institute's website noted that only 11 to 20 percent of people diagnosed with stage 4 inflammatory breast cancer live five or more years. In other words, it was unlikely that I would live five years.

But here I am ten years later, still working full time, traveling, and having lots of active adventures. I am doing well and, of course, I am still stage 4. I attribute this to palliative care. This extra layer of support helps with pain and symptom management, understanding my goals of care, spiritual support (there's even a chaplain on the team), and supporting my family and me.

You might be surprised to know that I did not choose a mastectomy (surgery to remove the breast) because the cancer is in every drop of blood in my body. The mastectomy would not remove the cancer and could cause me to have permanent swelling of my right arm, known as lymphadenopathy. I also don't take the most difficult combination chemotherapy regimens.

I had a discussion with my team about my goals. I said that I wanted a Niagara Falls trajectory. I felt good and wanted my care to focus on helping me to keep feeling good. But when I could no longer feel good, I did not want treatment to extend the bad days. So I wouldn't want an antibiotic if I was doing poorly and, say, developed pneumonia. If I had chosen the usual surgery and chemo-cocktails, it wouldn't cure me and would drop me off the cliff at day one. I chose the scenic route, my Niagara Falls scenic route.

Treatment

The medications I took were hormonal and for bone density. Over time, my medications have changed. I started on Femara and Zometa, and then was switched to Tamoxifen and Zometa. After that came Ibrance, Fasolodex and Xgeva. I am currently on two pills, Afinitor and Estemestane, with Xgeva injections, as well as calcium and vitamin D.

It hasn't always been smooth sailing, but palliative care has helped me avoid the problems that so many people encounter. For example, when the cancer spread to a new area of my spine it was very painful. The typical treatment is 10 to 20 doses of radiation, not to cure the cancer, just to get rid of the pain. My palliative care provider said a study of 16,000 people with cancer and painful bone metastases had just come out. It found that single fraction radiation—one larger dose of radiation— could be just as effective in addressing the pain. One dose would also mean less work missed, fewer side effects like fatigue, loss of appetite, and itching and peeling skin. But they also said sometimes you get a pain flare after treatment, meaning the pain gets worse before it goes away. So they gave me a pain medication I could take if that happened. "Pain meds can also cause terrible constipation, bad enough sometimes to cause you to end up in the emergency room," they said. They told me to take MiraLAX in addition if I needed to take the pain medication.

I often say that palliative care is the best friend of the seriously ill. My palliative care team helped me avoid unnecessary treatments that would have made me feel bad. They armed me with what I might need to avoid the emergency room. In the case of the painful bone mets, I had single-fraction radiation and the next day went to Washington, D.C.. I felt great. The pain was gone. I never got the pain flare. I never used the pain medication. My skin wasn't even red. Thank you, palliative care.

My Life Today

Since the diagnosis, I have gone on many adventures just like I did before cancer. I went reindeer sledding in the Arctic Circle last year, for example. I live a great life with inflammatory breast cancer, thanks to palliative care.

If you want to find the palliative care team in your community, go to www.getpalliativecare.org.

Part 3:
Afterword

Looking Ahead

Before the 1970s, long term survival with IBC was unlikely. Since then, however, there has been a steady improvement in the prognosis of newly diagnosed patients. We now understand that IBC is a systemic cancer with micro-metastases. That insight makes surgery and radiotherapy alone of limited use. Through advances in epidemiology, molecular biology, and treatment, we can predict how future improvements in outcome can be achieved.

In epidemiology, improvement in the case definition allowed doctors to recognize less dramatic clinical presentations of IBC. This clinical definition is now thus far similar to the Tunisian classification, where it was observed that patients with more limited clinical findings had the same profile and poor prognosis as patients with classic IBC.

As a result, the two primary U.S.-based organizations that recommend how IBC should be assessed and treated changed strategies. The NCI's Surveillance, Epidemiology and End Results Program revised coding to incorporate the expanded definition of IBC and update the prognosis data. This regrouping will allow researchers to identify subpopulations that are more heavily affected by IBC and find new risk factors for its development. The American Joint Committee on Cancer can now develop effective therapies based on experience and evidence in additional cases. In the new era of precision therapy, clinical trials that target molecular mechanisms are vital to advancement.

Molecular biology has identified markers and mechanisms that differentiate IBC from non-IBC breast cancer and show which mechanisms are susceptible to interruption by specific treatments. With more molecular biology tools, researchers are confident that they can identify cases of IBC early in their progression and offer specific treatments that will continue to improve breast cancer survival. In addition to identifying new IBC cases that have less than one-third of the breast clinically involved, molecular biology can examine if one type of rapidly progressing breast cancer–PEV1–is also part of the spectrum of IBC. If so, these patients would benefit from the same aggressive treatment that is used in IBC.

Molecular biology has not yet addressed the question of why some women have a much more dramatic response to initial combination chemotherapy than others. Could it be genetic resistance? Or differences in the gastrointestinal microbiome which may affect the metabolism of drugs they receive? Understanding this will be another step in improving IBC care.

Molecular biology also may lead to greater understanding of causation. The IBC Registry already has stored biospecimens from geographic clusters and family clusters including family members who are not genetically related, as in the case of a husband and wife with IBC, and it shares its samples with interested investigators. Although generally geographic studies focus on environment and family studies focus on genetics, looking at environmental triggers in non-genetically related family members is equally important. So far, genetics has not been shown to increase the likelihood of developing IBC or to affect survival, but the research goes on.

Molecular biology also contributes to treatment. Because it has identified the faulty gene that causes cystic fibrosis, it has enabled a new breakthrough treatment that targets the protein made by the gene, creating an effective treatment for 90 percent of the people with cystic fibrosis. Chronic myelocytic leukemia, which was considered untreatable twenty years ago, is now routinely controlled by drugs whose development was possible because researchers learned the molecular cause of the disease. The discovery of Herceptin as a treatment for patients with Her2-neu receptor positive breast cancer has been a major advance in the treatment of IBC and has shown significant therapeutic benefit.

The patient stories in this book provide important insights into the personal aspects of coping with IBC. Most important to the newly diagnosed patient is the message that long disease-free periods happen and they will be increasingly possible. It is even possible that this disease can be cured. Medical oncologists do not like to use the word "cure," but these stories do show long survivals which suggest the possibility of a cure. IBC survivors have stated various ways they have handled their treatments and used their post-treatment time to improve their lives. Some patients credit their faith for pulling them through. Some have focused on using their experience with IBC to propel them into careers as advocates: advising women newly diagnosed with breast cancer, serving as patient advocates for research proposals, and raising money for IBC and other forms of breast cancer. Their work has promoted awareness of IBC and an accurate understanding of IBC in the medical community, as well as in the general population. Some patients were never disease-free, yet enjoyed many years of productive happy lives even after their diagnoses. IBC was not a stumbling block but a stepping stone to a new and better life.

Among the many important lessons to take from the stories of these patients is that you must be your own strongest advocate. You know your body and what you need. If you are not happy with the medical advice or approach of your first doctor, get a second opinion, or even a third. There are too many possibilities for "right answers" for you not to be able to find the right path for you. One particularly instructive story emphasizes the potential of palliative care. Ten years after the patient was diagnosed, with that extra layer to help with pain and symptom management, provide spiritual support, and keep treatment focused on her individual goals of care, she still travels and works full time.

Another important lesson is that there is no discernable difference between long-term survivors and short-term survivors in their initial diagnosis, treatment, and ways of coping with IBC. This doesn't mean there are no reasons why some patients become long-term survivors—only that we haven't yet found them. Further research is essential to discovering these reasons so others may be helped. As treatment continues to evolve, we can expect improvements in IBC survival to continue. More than 180 patients have volunteered for study by the IBC Registry.

With their help and with that of new volunteers, we will offer new possibilities and hope for all patients with IBC.

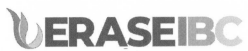

The Inflammatory Breast Cancer Foundation

EraseIBC is a grassroots non-profit that was formed to meet the dire need for education and research about inflammatory breast cancer. It was co-founded by Jenee Bobbora, an IBC survivor, Patti Bradfield, an IBC advocate and mother of Tina, who succumbed to the disease, and Dr. Massimo Cristofanilli (Dr. C), a renown IBC specialist and researcher. Our immediate goal was education because Dr. C was seeing so many cases of women who had been misdiagnosed due to lack of knowledge about the disease in the general public as well as in the medical community. We set out to develop materials that could be distributed, and we built a website with cutting-edge information about symptoms, diagnosis, and treatment.

Since its formation in 2007, EraseIBC has raised funds for educational materials, a website, and social media outreach, as well as for research. We were also instrumental in helping the first-ever clinic devoted to Inflammatory Breast Cancer get off the ground at MD Anderson in 2008. We help host small grassroots fundraisers and are proud of our biggest fundraiser to date, our inaugural IBC Impact Luncheon in 2015, which raised more than $240,000 for research at MD Anderson Cancer Center.

We are committed to educating people around the world and regularly send out materials to people who wish to help us in our mission. We have Girl Scouts who hand out pamphlets at meetings and we have booths at major medical conferences to ensure that young doctors and nurses are being made aware of the unusual presentation of IBC. We have hosted radio shows, held forums at major conferences, and sent volunteers out to speak in the community.

We invite you to join us in our mission. Please visit our website, EraseIBC.org, as well as our social media platforms. We want to completely erase the idea that all breast cancers present with a lump, and we want to help ensure that patients receive the most up-to-date treatment when they get diagnosed with IBC.

About the Authors

Paul H. Levine, MD

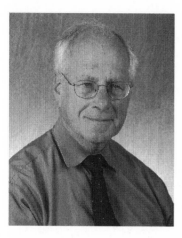

The experiences I have had in the almost 50 years studying IBC has brought me into contact with many talented people who have shaped my knowledge of the epidemiology of IBC and led to the development of the IBC Registry which has enrolled more than 180 patients.

This journey started in the early 1970s when Dr. Gregory O'Conor, then Director of the Fogarty International Center at NCI, introduced me to Dr. Dr. Nejib Mourali, the Director of the Institut Salah Azaiz (ISA) in Tunis. Dr. Mourali had been appointed as the first Director and organizer of ISA, the first Tunisian National Cancer Institute. With funds from the PL480 program which allowed countries benefiting from the PL480 Program, Tunisia was able to work with U.S. researchers to develop programs of interest to both countries and since IBC was a major problem in Tunisia with approximately 50 percent of breast cancer patients there diagnosed with IBC, that was an interesting challenge for a young epidemiologist like myself.

The work had to be done entirely in Tunisia with salaries paid in Tunisian dinars, so Dr. Mourali and I worked to get a multi-disciplinary team of Americans to work with his clinical and epidemiological staff to develop a laboratory at ISA and investigate the reason for this inordinately high incidence of IBC in Tunisia.

My summers in Tunisia provided an extraordinary experience and his clinical team led by Drs. Mourali and Francoise Tabbane, both surgeons, were doing breakthrough work developing one of the first neoadjuvant trials in IBC using three relatively inexpensive and available drugs, cyclophosphamide, methotrexate and 5-flurouracil (CMF) with excellent results in the first successful control of the disease there.

I saw more IBC patients in ISA each summer over the years than most medical oncologists see in a lifetime. When I moved from NCI to an academic career at The George Washington University, I decided to set up a Registry similar to one I had established at NCI for Burkitt's lymphoma (BL), a relatively rare U.S. malignancy similar to endemic BL in sub-Saharan Africa which was linked to the Epstein-Barr virus, the first human cancer virus investigated by NCI's Special Virus Leukemia Program.

I was given $10,000 by Owen Johnson's IBC Research Foundation to start this Registry. Owen's support and continuous help allowed us to recruit patients and obtain significant funding from the Dept. of Defense's Breast Cancer Program. That funding allowed the Registry to recruit colleagues and continue operation for more than 20 years, enrolling more than 180 patients.

The Registry, which supplied many research laboratories with biospecimens and very well documented clinical and epidemiologic data, owes its success to Carmela Veneroso, MPH, and Dr. Ladan Zolfaghari, who collected, organized, and inventoried the computerized and hard copy patient data and biospecimens, tracking the samples being distributed and helping to analyze the data. The large amount of information and research produced could only be possible with the hard work and dedication of the 180+ patients and their doctors, who were highly motivated to see their difficult experiences turn out to be beneficial to others facing IBC.

This book is the culmination of all those people who contributed to the Registry. Thank you all.

Deborah D. Lange

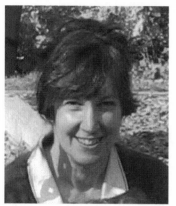

Deborah Lange is the president of Bethesda Communications Group, a publishing company, and is a teacher, writer, editor, and graphics designer living in Bethesda, MD. She has written on education and language change in national newspapers and journals, including her studies on why teenagers have led the change in the way we use word *like*. Her seminal research on this topic was published in *American Speech*. She holds degrees in English and linguistics.

She is the author of *Restoring the Glen Echo Park Carousel* and is a co-author with Richard Cook of *Glen Echo Park: A Story of Survival*. Bethesda Communications Group has previously published *Nobody's Listening: Stories of inflammatory Breast Cancer,* to which this book is a sequel.